MAYA

FIGHTING INFECTIONS SAVING LIVES

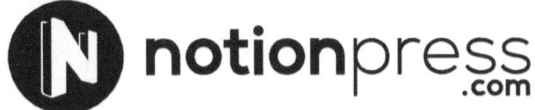

MAYA

FIGHTING INFECTIONS SAVING LIVES

KADIYALI M SRIVATSA

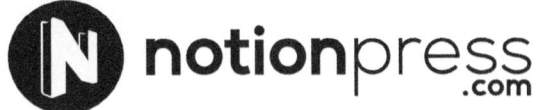

Notion Press

Old No. 38, New No. 6
McNichols Road, Chetpet
Chennai - 600 031

First Published by Notion Press 2016
Copyright © Kadiyali M Srivatsa 2016
All Rights Reserved.

ISBN 978-1-945497-89-6

This book has been published with all efforts taken to make the material error-free after the consent of the author. However, the author and the publisher do not assume and hereby disclaim any liability to any party for any loss, damage, or disruption caused by errors or omissions, whether such errors or omissions result from negligence, accident, or any other cause.

No part of this book may be used, reproduced in any manner whatsoever without written permission from the author, except in the case of brief quotations embodied in critical articles and reviews.

COMMON SYMPTOMS

1.	ABDOMINAL PAIN	3
2.	ALTERED STATE OF MIND	5
3.	AMENORRHOEA	6
4.	ANKLE PAIN	6
5.	ANKLE SWELLING	8
6.	APHASIA	9
7.	ARM NOT MOVING	10
8.	ARTHRALGIA	11
9.	ARTHRITIS	12
10.	ASCITES	13
11.	ASTHMA	14
12.	ASTHMATIC COUGH	15
13.	ATAXIA	16
14.	BABY CRYING WHEN FEEDING	19
15.	BACK PAIN	19
16.	BARKING COUGH	22
17.	BED WETTING	23
18.	BEHAVIORAL CHANGE	24
19.	BILE STAINED VOMITING	25
20.	BLEEDING AFTER SEX	25
21.	BLEEDING GUMS	26
22.	BLEEDING SPONTANEOUSLY	26

23.	BLOCKED NOSE	27
24.	BLOOD IN STOOLS	28
25.	BLOOD IN URINE	29
26.	BLOOD SHOT EYES	30
27.	BLUE COLORED FINGERS AND TOES	31
28.	BLURRED VISION	32
29.	BLUISH COLOR AROUND WOUND	33
30.	BOTH EYES ARE RED	33
31.	BREAST LUMP IN TEENAGER	34
32.	BREAST LUMP	34
33.	BREAST PAIN	36
34.	BREATHING DIFFICULTY IN ADULTS	37
35.	BREATHING DIFFICULTY IN CHILDREN	39
36.	BREATHING FAST	40
37.	BREATHLESSNESS WHEN SLEEPING	40
38.	BREATHLESSNESS WHEN WALKING UP HILL	41
39.	BREATHLESSNESS	42
40.	BREATHLESSNESS IN MERS AREA	43
41.	BRIGHT LIGHT HURTS THE EYE	44
42.	BURNING SENSATION WHEN PASSING URINE	45
43.	BUZZING NOISE IN EARS	47
44.	CANCER	48
45.	CANNOT BEAR TO SEE BRIGHT LIGHT	49
46.	CHEST PAIN	49
47.	CHEST PAIN WHEN BREATHING IN	51
48.	CHESTY COUGH	51

49.	CHICKEN POX	53
50.	CHICKEN POX RASH	54
51.	CHILLS AND RIGORS	55
52.	CHOKING	56
53.	CIRCULAR ITCHY RASH	56
54.	CIRCULAR NON-ITCHY RASH	57
55.	COLD	58
56.	COLD AND SHIVERING	59
57.	COLD SORE	60
58.	CONFUSION	61
59.	CONJUNCTIVITIS	62
60.	CONTACT LENS STUCK IN EYE	63
61.	CONVULSIONS	64
62.	CORNS AND CALLUSES	65
63.	COUGH - BARKING TYPE	67
64.	COUGH – DRY	68
65.	COUGHING AFTER EXERCISE	69
66.	COUGHING AT NIGHT	70
67.	COUGHING EVERY MORNING	72
68.	COUGHING IN ASTHMA	74
69.	COUGHING IN CHILDREN	76
70.	COUGHING IN MERS	77
71.	COUGHING OUT BLOOD	79
72.	COUGHING OUT FRESH BLOOD	79
73.	COUGHING OUT GREEN PHLEGM	80
74.	CRADLE CAP	81

75.	CROUPY COUGH	82
76.	CRYING BABY	84
77.	CRYING BABY DURING FLYING	85
78.	CYSTITIS	86
79.	DELIRIOUS	87
80.	DIABETES	88
81.	DIARRHOEA IN MERS	89
82.	DIARRHOEA WATERY	90
83.	DIARRHOEA WITH BLOOD	92
84.	DIARRHOEA AFTER RETURNING FROM HOLIDAY	93
85.	DIARRHOEA IN EBOLA ENDEMIC AREA	94
86.	DIFFICULT TO BREATHE	95
87.	DYSARTHRIA	96
88.	DISCHARGE FROM PENIS OR VAGINS	96
89.	DISMENNORHOEA	98
90.	DIZZINESS	99
91.	DOG BITE	100
92.	DOUBLE VISION	101
93.	DRINKING MORE WATER	101
94.	DROWSINESS	102
95.	DRY EYE	103
96.	DRY MOUTH	104
97.	DRY SKIN	105
98.	DYSENTERY	106
99.	DYSPHAGIA	107
100.	DYSUREA	108

101.	EAR WITH WATERY DISCHARGE	109
102.	ECZEMA	110
103.	EYE HARD	112
104.	EYE IS RED	113
105.	EYE ITCHY	114
106.	EYE STICKY	115
107.	EYELID HAS A LUMP	116
108.	EYES ARE WATERY	117
109.	EYES LOOK YELLOW	118
110.	EYES PAIN	119
111.	EYES WITH FLOATERS	119
112.	FAINTING	120
113.	FALL	122
114.	FATIGUE	123
115.	FEELING COLD	124
116.	FEELING HOT AND COLD	125
117.	FEELING LOW	126
118.	FEVER	128
119.	FEVER AND FITS	130
120.	FEVER IS MODERATE	131
121.	FEVER Temp 36–38°C or 98–100°F	132
122.	FEVER VERY HIGH	133
123.	FITS	134
124.	FLUSH - FEELING OR LOOK FLUSHED	135
125.	FLU	136
126.	FOUL SMELLING VAGINAL DISCHARGE	137
127.	FRESH BLOOD IN STOOL	138

128.	GASTRIC ULCER	138
129.	GASTRITIS	139
130.	GENITAL BLISTERS	140
131.	GERMAN MEASLES (Rubella)	141
132.	GREEN COLORED (BILE VOMIT)	142
133.	HANGOVER	142
134.	HEAD ACHE	143
135.	HEAD INJURY	145
136.	HEAD LICE	146
137.	HEART BURN	147
138.	HEAT RASH	148
139.	HIGH PITCHED CRY	150
140.	HOARSE VOICE	151
141.	HOT AND SWEATY	152
142.	IMPETIGO	152
143.	IMPOTENCY	153
144.	INDIGESTION	154
145.	INJURY MINOR	155
146.	INJURY SEVERE	156
147.	INSECT BITE	156
148.	INSOMNIA	157
149.	IRRITABILITY	159
150.	IRRITABLE BOWEL	160
151.	ITCHING AFTER HOT BATH	162
152.	ITCHY ANUS	162
153.	ITCHY LUMPS ON LEGS AND ARMS	163

154.	ITCHY PENIS	164
155.	ITCHY RASH	165
156.	ITCHY VAGINA	166
157.	ITCHY AFTER HOT BATH	167
158.	JAUNDICE	167
159.	KIDNEY STONES	168
160.	KNEE PAIN	169
161.	LEG PAIN AND SWELLING	169
162.	LEGS NOT MOVING	170
163.	LIGHT HURTS CHILDS EYE	172
164.	LIPS ARE BLUE	172
165.	LOSS OF APPETITE	173
166.	LOSS OF CONCENTRATION	173
167.	LUMP – RED HOT PAINFUL	174
168.	LUMP IN ANAL REGION	174
169.	LUMP IN GROIN	175
170.	LUMP ON EYE LID	176
171.	MEASLES	176
172.	MEMORY LOSS	178
173.	MENINGITIS	179
174.	MERS, Middle East Respiratory Syndrome	180
175.	MIGRAINE	181
176.	MISCARRAIGE	182
177.	MUMPS	183
178.	NAPPY RASH	185
179.	NAUSEA	186

180.	NECK PAIN	186
181.	NETTLE RASH	187
182.	NO FEVER	188
183.	NO OTHER SYMPTOM	188
184.	NOISY BREATHING	189
185.	NOSE BLEEDING	190
186.	NOSE BLOCKED	191
187.	NUMBNESS	192
188.	OFFENSIVE DISCHARGE	192
189.	PAINFUL PERIODS	192
190.	PAIN IN ABDOMEN	193
191.	PAIN AND LUMP IN THROAT	195
192.	PAIN AND SWELLING AFTER A FALL	195
193.	PAIN IN BOTH EARS	196
194.	PAIN IN ONE EAR	197
195.	PAIN IN TESTES	198
196.	PAIN IN VAGINA	199
197.	PAIN IN VAGINA DURING AND AFTER SEX	200
198.	PAIN WORSE WHEN CLIMBING UP	201
199.	PAIN WORSE WHILE CLIMBING DOWN	202
200.	PAINFUL ANKLE	203
201.	PAINFUL LUMP IN ANUS	203
202.	PALPITATIONS	204
203.	PASSING LESS URINE	205
204.	PASSING MORE URINE	206
205.	PERIOD PAINS	207

206.	PELVIC INFECTION	207
207.	PEPTIC ULCER	208
208.	PERIODS IRREGULAR	209
209.	PERIODS MISSED	210
210.	PHOTOPHOBIA	211
211.	POISONING	212
212.	POLYUREA	213
213.	POOR HEARING	214
214.	POST-MENOPAUSAL BLEEDING,	215
215.	PREMATURE EJACULATION	215
216.	PREGNANCY	216
217.	RAPID WEIGHT GAIN,	217
218.	RASH COMES AND GOES	219
219.	RASH ITCHY	220
220.	RASH ITCHY AFTER HOT BATH	220
221.	RASH LOOKS LIKE CHICKEN POX	221
222.	RASH DOES NOT DISAPPEAR WITH PRESSURE	222
223.	RED COLORED RASH	222
224.	RED OR PURPLE RASH	223
225.	RED RASH	223
226.	REDUCED VISION	224
227.	RETURNED FROM HOLIDAY	224
228.	RING WORM	225
229.	RUNNY NOSE	226
230.	SCABIES	227
231.	SEPTICEMIA	228

232.	SHINGLES	230
233.	SKIN IS YELLOW	231
234.	SNEEZING EXCESSIVE	232
235.	SOILING IN BED	233
236.	SQUINT	234
237.	STOOLS BLACK OR TARRY	234
238.	STRUGGLING TO BREATHEE	235
239.	SWELLING AROUND JAW	236
240.	SWELLING AROUND WOUND	237
241.	SWELLING IN THE NECK	237
242.	SWOLLEN LEGS	238
243.	SWOLLEN TESTES	238
244.	SWOLLEN TUMMY	239
245.	SWALLOWING DIFFICULTY	239
246.	TALKING FUNNY	240
247.	THROAT HAS WHITE SPOTS	240
248.	THROAT LUMP	241
249.	THRUSH IN MOUTH	241
250.	TINGLING SENSATION	242
251.	TINNITUS	242
252.	TRAVEL SICKNESS	243
253.	TUMMY BLOATING	245
254.	TUMMY PAIN	246
255.	UNABLE TO BREATH	247
256.	UNABLE TO SEE BRIGHT LIGHT	248
257.	UNABLE TO SLEEP	248

258.	UNABLE TO SPEAK	250
259.	UNCONSCIOUSNESS	252
260.	UNPROTECTED SEX	253
261.	URINE – BURNING SENSATION	255
262.	URTICARIAL RASH	256
263.	VAGINAL BLEEDING	257
264.	VAGINAL PAIN DURING SEX	257
265.	VAGINAL THRUSH	258
266.	VERTIGO	259
267.	VISION SUDDEN LOSS OF VISION	261
268.	VOMITING	262
269.	VOMITING AFTER BOUT OF COUGH	262
270.	VOMITING BLOOD	263
271.	WART	263
272.	WEAKNESS	264
273.	WEAKNESS IN ONE SIDE OF BODY	265
274.	WHEEZING	265
275.	WHEEZY COUGH	266
276.	WHITE DISCHARGE FROM GENITALIA	267
277.	WHITE DISCHARGE FROM VAGINA	268
278.	WHITE SPOTS IN MOUTH	269
279.	WHOOPING COUGH	270
280.	WIND OR FLATULENCE	271
281.	WRIST PAIN	273

PREFACE

It's not long since I heard stories about clinical errors committed by Dr Sullman, working as a junior doctor in the early 1990s that made me shudder with fright. "That could have been me working as a junior doctor in Christie's hospital, Manchester," in the 1980s. He had the worst experience not because he was a bad doctor, but due to an organizational error and vital information about administering the drug, that had gone.

Serious murders committed by Dr Harold Shipman must have shocked institutions and angered every doctor working in them in early 2000. A majority of us blamed the institutions, and now I have reason to believe these institutions are responsible for what is going on in the healthcare, and why doctors like me find it blame unjustly.

Much of Britain's legal structure concerning health care and medicine is said to have been reviewed and modified as a result of Shipman's crimes. Dr Sullman spoke publicly about the problem of working as a junior doctor in the hospitals and said things still haven't changed in the National Health Service (NHS). He is right, because the problems in the NHS are not as simple or straightforward as explained above.

To understand why, how and what is going on in the medical profession, you must be a qualified doctor, pass examinations to prove you are safe to examine, diagnose and treat fellow humans as patients. To master the art of clinical medicine, you must work with critically ill adults and children in hospital for almost twenty to thirty years.

After reading various books written by doctors, patients and following news about disease, illness and advances in healthcare published in medical journals and media, doctors like us start feeling very uncomfortable. Over-enthusiastic urge to encourage consultations, perform investigations, hospitalization, operations and prescribing drugs that may or may not be necessary has tarnished the image of our profession.

Knowing and understanding how doctors think, act and behave is complex because the information they have is very confidential. A doctor will find it hard to raise concerns about wrong doings knowing that the General Medical Council will prosecute him for breaching confidentiality and he will be ostracized.

After mastering the art of clinical diagnosis, and the management of complex illnesses in adults and children we developed a simple tool. In 2003 we created MAYA (Medical Advice You Access) to help receptionists, nurses, doctors in training and patients to differentiate minor from serious illnesses.

Knowing Antibiotic Resistant Bacteria and viral infections not only threaten our profession but also our very existance. We feel seeking alternatives to fight infections is very essential. Finding eighteen new antibiotics to fight an army of micro-organisms is likely to remain a dream. The only option we have to help reduce the threat is to identify infected patients early, isolate and prevent them from spreading their infection in our community and hospitals.

In 2006, we shared this information with people in power, members of the nursing profession (nurse practitioners and prescribers) who were made to work as primary care physicians in the NHS. We were not aware this simple tool that could be shared using advances in communication technology would indeterminate our passion.

After enduring ten years of harassment, humiliation and struggles, we have published this book to share our experience and knowledge to help protect humanity. We sincerely hope our contribution will directly or indirectly bring tears of happiness that will make us feel proud and happy.

We thank you for purchasing our book, subscribing to our website and using our apps to learn how to differentiate minor from serious illness. We hope to use the symptoms you log in to identify infected individuals and isolate them to help protect families and the community and to avert epidemics that may happen in the future.

We are challenging the institutions that have been inflicting pain and suffering on fellow human beings who trust doctors by offering sub'standard medical service, performing unnecessary investigations and abusing antibiotics.

FUTURE PANDEMICS & EPIDEMICS

In the article published (The most predictable disaster in the history of the human race by Ezra Klien) on May 27, 2015, named "The most predictable threat in the history of the human race," Bill Gates said "No one can say we weren't warned." And warned. And warned. A pandemic disease is the most predictable catastrophe in the history of the human race, if only because it has happened to the human race so many, many times before. He found out more people died after the First World War as a result of Spanish flu in the 1920's than the total who died in World War I & II combined.

Infectious diseases claimed more lives than all wars, non-infectious diseases, and natural disasters put together. Infectious diseases were our oldest, deadliest foes in the pre-antibiotic era and have now rapidly become a major threat to humanity. Year after year, we hear about infections killing people in thousands and spreading from one country to another, but not many have developed a strategy to stop this happen.

WHY?

In 2014–15, it was the Ebola infection which killed more than 10,000 people. As we predicted, spreading infection is not only a threat to humanity but a threat to our profession, (TV Interview broadcasted in Sky 4 in Suriname). More than fifty per cent (50%) of people who died were healthcare workers (doctors, nurses, lab technicians, ambulance staff and workers).

In 2015, a particularly infectious form of bird flu ripped through fourteen states, forcing public healthcare workers to enforce the slaughter of 39 million birds in USA. The result of such a callous act has made viruses and bacteria mutate and reassemble themselves into a form which can now infect humans.

It isn't just the news that carries warnings, but the fear of infectious disease exists in every person's mind. Until now no one has come forward to join hands and help us develop strategies to educate, share knowledge to help people identify and prevent the spread of infection in their family and community. The majority of stakeholders have been obstructive to disruptive technologies we have developed to help reduce the spread of these infections.

We invented ET Tube holders, to help reduce accidental extubations to reduce multiple intubations, U-Cannula to help reduce the number of multiple attempts and MAYA to reduce access to healthcare because we believe that slowing down the spread of MRSA (Methicillin Resistant Staph Abreus) in hospitals is mandatory to reduce the threat to humanity. Our mission was to reduce cross infections and the abuse of antibiotics. Unfortunately, we had no choice but to develop disruptive innovations because scientists and pharmaceutical companies have not developed a simple cost effective method to help reduce the spread of infections in the community or hospitals.

We spoke to scientists, agencies and pharmaceutical companies at the Superbug Super Drug conference in London. They are only insisting and talking about investing millions of dollars to help them invent another antibiotic, tests and test hypothesis, claiming this to be the way forward.

Dr Lloyd Czaplewski in his presentation "What if there are no new antibiotics? Highlights of a Wellcome Trust & Department of Health (England)" initiated and sponsored a review and report into "Alternatives to Antibiotics." He did not list preventive strategies using Internet or communication software to help reduce the spread of infections in families, community and countries.

Various hypotheses and strategies to fight infections were discussed but they still think vaccination is the only option to help prevent infections and reduce spread. Knowing there are hundreds of bacteria, viruses and fungi requiring drugs to kill them, how can we even contemplate to fight the threat from an army of micro-organisms we have not yet encountered?

The microbiologists and pharmacologists say that it would take at least ten years before one antibiotic (Phase I trial) can reach the market, costing billions of dollars, yet with no guarantee of developing and marketing treatments to fight infections. The group formed by European Commission are not spending time or money to help develop methods to identify infected individuals or to manage infected patients and reduce spread.

HISTORY OF THREE DECADES OF INFECTIONS

In 1980s "AIDS" was given more importance because this affected some rich and famous people. Spreading MRSA in hospitals was ignored. We anticipated bacterial threat will bring us to our knees and kill millions of people worldwide, but device and equipment manufacturers and pharmaceutical companies ignored our concern. They continued to highlight needle phobia and spread of HIV infections to healthcare workers and ignored the fact that thousands of patients were dying in hospital as a result of MRSA.

Antibiotic resistant infection in hospital went from an obscure hospital problem to a global pandemic. This, alongside emerging infections has become the most common cause of death in the world. One bacteria has now shared its knowledge and technical know-how with other bacteria, viruses and even fungi.

The CDC has released a document titled "Preparedness 101 Zombie Apocalypse." They said they do not expect a zombie apocalypse to be around the corner; but say educating people to avoid becoming a zombie will help make them aware of spreading a pandemic of infectious disease.

When we discuss this topic, doctors, nurses and people shut down, and so no one plans for an actual crisis as it is just too scary and too paralyzing to think about.

Pandemic disease is something we talk about when it happens rather than before and then we forget about it as soon as the threat wanes off. The healthcare professionals think about it, know about it and are afraid. As doctors, this is in our minds and haunts us in our nightmares, but we cannot even talk to people who work in healthcare because they are too scared to talk about it.

We think about it so much. It seems almost ridiculous that we aren't ready and still not even contemplating the "Threat to humanity and our profession is real" and so we're not ready, and not even close to even start thinking about it.

Ebola infection has now made some healthcare workers understand what we are talking about and so it's getting easier, but we feel this will not get us far.

Americans ignored the advice of WHO taking eight months to make the information public, resulting in healthcare workers dying in their thousands of Ebola. Americans and Europeans were used to hearing stories about epidemics and pandemics and assumed this to be someone else's problem.

Ebola is very difficult to transmit because people who are contagious have visible symptoms. It broke out in three relatively small countries which don't send many travellers to the US. Those three countries have good relationships with America and were welcoming of western aid.

In the future we anticipate emerging infections and pandemic flu which kills millions will not have visible symptoms. It could break out in a highly populous country that sends thousands of travellers a day all over the world. It could be in a country with huge population like India, China and Africa and in countries and areas which are not easily accessible.

The world is not prepared to deal with infectious diseases which can spread across the world faster than Spanish flu, even though it's been known about for decades and we have seen how people have died in the past.

A person infected with a contagious disease can expect to pass the disease on to two people. This is called the "reproduction number."

Two is not that high a number, as these things go. The SARS virus had a reproduction number of four. Measles has a reproduction number of eighteen.

One person travelling as a passenger and carrying an infection similar to Ebola or Viral infection can infect three to five people sitting around him and ten if he walks to the toilet. The study was conducted and published in a medical journal a few years ago, but the airline industry has not implemented changes or introduced screening to prevent spreading infections.

Nobody knows what will happen when the world faces a lethal disease we're not used to with a reproduction number of five or eight or even ten. What if it starts in a megacity? What if, unlike Ebola, it's contagious before the patient is showing obvious symptoms?

Past experience isn't comforting. "H1N1 flu in 2009, had spread around the world before we even knew it existed."

THE PROBLEMS

Countries will not admit they have a problem and request help because of the possible financial implications. They don't want to admit they have a problem because in terms of investors and travel, it's a death sentence.

Guinea did not declare the Ebola epidemic; Chinese leaders, worried about trade and tourism and lied about the presence of the virus for months in 2002. In 2004, when avian influenza first surfaced in Thailand, officials there displayed a similar reluctance to release information.

Hospitals in countries like India are managed and often owned by doctors. They refuse to share information about existing infections and categorically decline to accept they have a problem. Reporting infections to public health authorities is not mandatory. Doctors and hospitals who fail to report are not penalized. Even now the WHO or CDC do not have information about spreading E. Coli or other infections.

Countries like Syria or Yemen are weak and fragmented to effectively co- ordinate and are hostile to organizations which would need to come in and offer relief.

A third problem is that the majority of poor nations do not trust the efficacy of the international institutions and will not co-ordinate or co-operate with agencies.

The World Health Organization's Ebola performance was a disaster. There was slow response to declare a public health emergency even some five months after public warnings from Frontieres (Doctors Without Borders), doctors were on the front line when they died.

This isn't just an issue of bureaucratic incompetence. The WHO is underpowered for the problems it's meant to solve. Funding comes from voluntary donations, and there's no mechanism by which it can quickly scale up its efforts during an emergency.

The result is that the WHO that will face the next major disease outbreak is likely to be quite similar to the WHO that faced Ebola, and H1N1, and SARS.

Stakeholders admit we need another mechanism. Most experts agree that the world needs some kind of emergency-response team for dangerous diseases, but no one knows quite how to set up that team.

This is in stark contrast to war, which is not necessarily more deadly to the human race, but is much better planned for. There are a wealth of rules regarding how the government can seize various ships, yet when an epidemic arrives, who is supposed to survey the private capacity and go out there and grab all these things?

We do not have an equivalent of the military reserve, where you get on the phone and mobilize a team of experts to contain infections. People who want to volunteer are not paid. What do we do with them after they have returned, when people might have this fear that they've been exposed to infection? Are employers going to take them back? What are the quarantine rules? It is completely ad hoc. Unlike in previous eras, humanity does not have the tools it needs to protect itself.

Global travel has far outpaced global governance or even global disease response. Diseases move much faster than governments. We are not prepared and no one really knows how to fix it.

HOW WE HELP MICRO-ORGANISMS TO SPREAD

Behind Gates' fear of pandemic disease is an algorithmic model of how disease moves through the modern world. He initially funded that model to help with his foundation's work eradicating polio, but then he used it to consider how a disease which acted like the Spanish flu of 1918 would work in today's world.

The results even shocked Mr Gates. His model predicted that the spread of infection in all urban centers around the entire globe can occur in sixty days. The basic reason why the disease could spread fifty times faster is that human beings now move around and cross borders today much more than they did in 1918.

And any new disease will cross those borders with them and will do so before we necessarily even know such a new disease exists. According to Bill Gates' model, a Spanish flu-like disease would kill more than 33 million people in 250 days.

"We've created, in terms of spread, the most dangerous environment that we've ever had in the history of mankind," Gates says.

Underdeveloped health systems threaten developed countries. According to the World Health Organization, the United States spends more than $8,000 per person, per year, on health care. Eritrea spends less than $20.

Politicians and health decision makers consider that to be Eritrea's problem but if a highly infectious, highly lethal new disease presents in Eritrea, and the world is slow to learn about it, then it will quickly become the world's problem.

If Ebola had made its first appearance in the United States or Europe it would have been caught, and contained quickly. However, this outbreak began in three of the poorest countries in the world, and it took them at least three months to even realize they were harboring an Ebola outbreak. By the time Ebola was recognized, it was already out of control and so, for the first time, it made its way to American shores.

We must halt the spread of infectious diseases early and implement the most effective way to protect people. It is not the basic public health infrastructure, laboratories, finding specimens, tests to discover what's spreading, but offering a simple tool to help people share information about their clinical symptoms and using sophisticated software to monitor them.

Emergency operation centers, infectious disease control centers and doctors will be informed after identifying clusters of similar symptoms. This will help mobilize services to isolate infected individuals and prevent them from travelling to healthcare centers or emergency rooms in hospitals, spreading their infection as they travel and to patients and healthcare workers in the hospitals.

The good news about our system is that it's not expensive, it's ready to go live and can be shared using Internet technology. We have identified local doctors with the help of people living in the area and formed a network of people, local doctors and healthcare centers to help monitor and organize the management of infections.

By allowing doctors to create a database of symptoms using their local language we hope to help protect healthcare workers and people. We have spent years thinking, testing and developing a tool which is simple to use and not expensive to implement.

Basic public health infrastructure is fairly cheap – around a dollar per person, per year. Uganda may have motorcycle couriers picking up specimens from hundreds and hundreds of health care centers all over the country but their lives are at risk and so the system may collapse. Sending specimens to centralized centers is useful if we have tests and methods to identify the organisms, but we don't have a single test which can diagnose all the infectious disease. Emerging bacteria and viruses have mutated and so they are difficult to detect.

The difficulty often isn't money; it's prioritizing services, communication, delegating responsibility and implementing changes in law so that people and healthcare providers report symptoms and seek help early.

If we can find the disease and have a test to diagnose it, then modern technology really does help, but if we cannot diagnose infection and have no tests available to identify infecting organisms, we have a major problem to manage.

Scientists believe they can rapidly decode the basic structure and pathways of new diseases in ways that were unimaginable even a few decades ago. They claim to have come up with a much more rapid response, but this relies on patients coming forward to say they have a symptom which may require investigating and treatment. We know from our past experience that patients with serious symptoms are often in denial and ignore it until it's too late. The reason they do not seek help from doctors is because they do not want doctors to confirm their fear.

I was called to see a passenger during a flight. The history presented to me by a member of the cabin crew was typical of infection. To tell you frankly, I was scared to see this passenger knowing all about infections like Ebola spreading in Africa. This made me worry and so I developed a simple solution which could screen passengers before they boarded the flight.

We know that passengers travelling from a country with spreading infections that kill, will not be honest to admit they have a symptom that suggests infection. We have no method that could swiftly communicate and block travellers boarding flights and spreading the infection back in their home town.

We are sure [the WHO] will not do better next time because this organization is too big and complicated to handle a future crisis. We must think and act now to avert a tsunami of infection that will wipe out a generation.

By offering help to people by allowing them to download Dr MAYA, FREE of cost, offering advice to help manage basic health care, we can develop a monitor that identifies clusters of infection in hospitals, community, town or country. Offering a tool to help doctors communicate, manage their patients better and reduce cost of running their clinic or office will encourage them to participate.

This tool was developed and managed by a doctor who was subjected to harassment for defending patients' care in the UK for ten years. He developed the tool initially to help protect fellow humans and reduce medical errors, cross infections, cost and antibiotic abuse.

Using the same tool and creating an APP for doctors to create their own Dr MAYA, he has made it possible to initially identify infected individuals and isolate them by sharing information with the doctor. The lives of doctors, nurses, staff and family will be protected by preventing patients from visiting them, and it is likely to be accepted and used to help us fight a major threat to humanity.

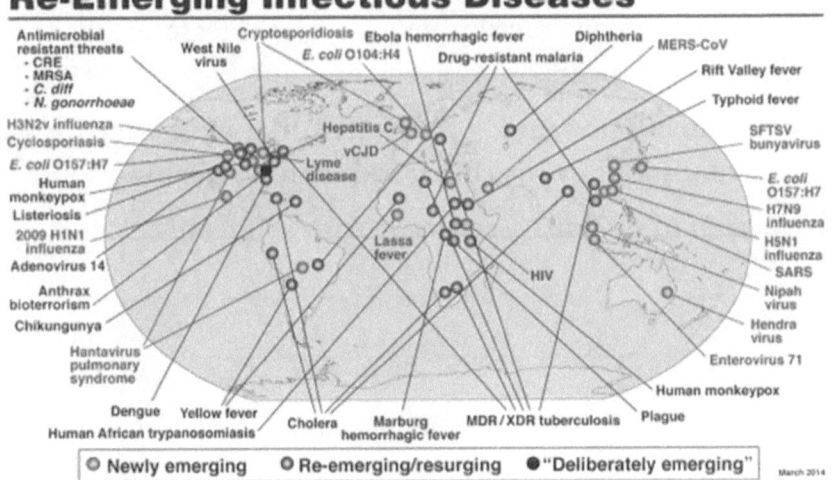

INFORMATION

The content we have provided in this book or App is the general information that doctors working in hospitals and community provide. The symptoms and diseases listed are common illnesses that make you very anxious and you rush to consult a doctor. Using our App, you will learn about the symptoms and illnesses that are associated, so that you will know what and why you may need tests, investigations or take specific treatment. This should not be treated as a substitute for the medical advice offered by your doctor.

We do not endorse any commercial product, religious organization, political organization, healthcare providers, institution or service providers. We may share information or support NGOs or institutions that are striving hard to make life better for the sick and vulnerable.

Please consult your own GP, doctors or specialist if you're in any way concerned about your baby's or your health. We sincerely hope you will find our contribution very helpful. Please email us your comments, compliments or criticize our effort.

As a wise man once said, "The only thing necessary for the triumph of evil is that good men do nothing".

Dedicated to students, parents, friends and family.

BRING BACK THE LOST HUMAN FACE OF MEDICINE.

MAYA is a "tool" and not a medical textbook or a book you use to learn a new skill or acquire knowledge. The information provided in this book is based on how experienced doctors arrive at a diagnosis to offer advice and treatment.

You should not read this book in the same way as you read a novel or a book which teaches you how to develop personal skills. Although you must familiarize yourself with the list of symptoms, do not go through the notes and information if you are well. If you do this, it is possible to become paranoid and start imagining that you have some of these illnesses.

If you are not feeling well, or have any specific symptoms, please use our App, book, or website, and go through the information provided there.

The color chart will either prompt or discourage you to go to hospital, demand an emergency appointment or consult doctors. If the combination of symptoms suggests a minor illness, MAYA will advise you to consult either a nurse or a pharmacist at the local chemist's.

If you do not find your symptoms here, please speak to a doctor, or in case of emergency, consult or go directly to a hospital. You can find information about individual symptoms using Google or other search engines.

DOCTORS' DUTY, ETHICS AND SERVICE TO HUMANITY

Experienced doctors will not use flow charts, protocols, algorithms, or pocket books of differential diagnoses to help them manage any illness. They know that when patients describe the symptoms for which they require professional attention, they are reporting the story of an illness they have lived as they remember it, and so it can vary. To some extent, symptoms are a universal human experience as virtually every person experiences some discomfort.

Labeling an illness based on symptoms (wheezy bronchitis, sore throat, chesty cough, flu-like illness, red ears or red throat) or naming a disease using Latin, Greek or other languages (Arthritis, pneumonitis, pharyngitis) is not the most important factor which differentiates a good doctor from the bad ones.

A doctor working in primary care, or in the jungles of Borneo, or a remote village in the Himalayas, does not have access to sophisticated equipment, tests and drugs. If he or she "does something which another doctor in a similar situation will not do" or "does not do something which another doctor in similar situation would have done," he or she will be criticized as being "negligent" (Alderson 1843).

Since 2003, we have identified numerous clinical errors committed by doctors and nurses working in primary care. As doctors working in primary care, we started identifying more patients returning to consult us with minor or serious complications. We identified numerous clinical errors in diagnosis, advice and treatment offered to patients.

Minor and serious complications occurred because given a similar situation we would have made the right diagnosis and offered the correct treatment, or not offered a wrong diagnosis and treatment resulting in prolonged pain with the patient suffering devastating consequences.

We would have referred some patients to hospital early when the combination of common symptoms suggested a potentially serious illness which could result in long-term complications, or even death. The majority of doctors and nurses all over the world provide their patients with good care, but a few are committing serious errors which bring shame upon us all.

Unfortunately, patients and relatives who have suffered, find it difficult to prove clinical negligence, as it is not always a straightforward process. Knowing how we struggle to defend our ethics and profession to protect humanity, we know people in power are using the legal system and the so-called evidence based medicine to conceal the truth.

MAYA was developed based on research and clinical acumen used by doctors working in acute and intensive care for almost thirty years. We have admitted, discharged and referred adults and children to go back to their GP (family doctor) using the same criteria and have unblemished registration to work in UK.

The World Medical Association Tokyo Declaration states, "A doctor must have complete clinical independence in deciding the care of a person for whom he or she is medically responsible. The doctor's fundamental role is to alleviate the distress of his or her fellow men, and no motive, whether personal, collective, or political, shall prevail against this higher purpose."

HEALTH CARE IN INDIA

Now the problem of unethical medical practice, increased privatization and the problem of offering services using medically untrained persons and nurses has been highlighted.

In India, private medical schools funded by private investors, religious organizations, and doctors were established in the last twenty years. These schools offer to train students who pay enormous amounts of donations and fees. The quality of training is likely to be not very high due to the shortage of very experienced clinicians as teachers

After qualification, doctors often establish multi-specialty hospitals offering healthcare to Indians and people from other countries.

Medical tourism is a growing in business sector in India. In October 2015, India's medical tourism sector was estimated to be worth US$3 billion and projected to grow to $7–8 billion by 2020. The primary reason that attracts patients is cost-effectiveness. It offers wide variety of procedures at about one-tenth the cost of similar procedures in the United States.

Foreign patients travelling to India to seek medical treatment in 2012, 2013 and 2014 numbered 171,021, 236,898, and 184,298 respectively (*Press Information Bureau*. Retrieved 28 April 2016)

The cost of healthcare has increased, resulting in more than 90% of patients admitted to hospital in India, 700,000 in USA and 400,000 in UK being bankrupted. This inflicts pain and suffering on families, and so is unethical.

Nearly three-quarters of doctors request lab tests, perform procedures, refer patients, and offer specific treatments, in order to boost their own income. Even knowing that our profession is now threatened by antibiotic resistant bacterial infections, doctors are still living under an illusion. They are reluctant to implement changes to defend our ethics and help protect humanity.

HISTORY OF MEDICINE

Early medical traditions include those of ancient Egypt and Babylon where healthcare originated. The Greeks introduced the concepts of medical diagnosis, prognosis, and medical ethics. The "Hippocrates Oath," first written in the 5th century BC, Greece, has been significantly changed by doctors in the 19th century, but is still accepted today.

In the medieval ages, surgical practices inherited from the ancient masters were improved and then systematized in *The Practice of Surgery*. Universities formally established a system to train physicians around the year 1220 in Italy.

During the Renaissance period, the understanding of human anatomy improved, and the microscope was invented. The "germ theory of disease" was accepted in the 19th century. Military doctors advanced the methods of trauma treatment and surgery. Public health measures were developed, especially in the 19th century as the rapid growth of cities required systematic sanitary measures in UK and Europe.

Advanced research centers opened in the early 20th century, often connected with major hospitals. The mid-20th century was characterized by new biological treatments, such as antibiotics. These advancements, along with developments in chemistry, genetics, and lab technology, such as the X-Ray, led to modern medicine.

Medicine was heavily professionalized in the 20th century. New careers opened up to women as nurses, starting in the 1870s, and as physicians, especially after 1970. The 21st century is characterized by highly advanced research involving numerous fields of science.

DISCOVERY OF PENICILLIN

In 1895, Vincenzo Tiberio, an Italian researcher and medical officer of the Medical Corps of the Italian Navy and physician at the University of Naples, noticed that the people who drank water from a well after they had removed the mould from the wall of the well complained of severe abdominal pain and intestinal upset.

He published a paper, "The antibacterial power of some extracts of mould (Penicillium glaucum)," making him the discoverer of the antibacterial property of penicillin. At the time, his work was disregarded as coincidence and received no further support or recognition.

A French physician, Ernest Duchesne, of Lyon, France, published a medical thesis, "Contribution to the study in vital competition in micro-organisms: antagonism between moulds and microbes," in 1897. He began testing the effect of French tap water on mould and discovered that mould significantly inhibited bacterial growth. He discovered that the presence of Penicillium glaucum in tap water worked like an antibiotic. Duchesne understood the therapeutic effect of this mould in animals and demonstrated how extracts from Penicillium glaucum saved dying guinea pigs.

Because he was just twenty-three years old and unknown, the Pasteur Institute did not acknowledge receipt of his dissertation and published information. They called for more research, but unfortunately, his army service prevented him from doing any further work. Neither Duchesne nor the Pasteur Institute capitalized on this amazing discovery.

Twenty-eight years later, Clodomiro Picado Twight, a Costa Rican scientist born in Nicaragua, became a pioneer in the research of snakes, serpent venoms, and the development of various antivenins. His work on moulds was a precursor to the formal discovery of penicillin. In 1923, he showed how a group of fungi of the "penicillin" genre inhibited the growth of staphylococci. His work resulted in compounds, which he used to treat patients at least one year before the commonly accepted discovery of penicillin.

Thirty-three years after Vincenzo Tiberio's discovery and five years after Clodomiro Picado Twight demonstrated the inhibition of Staphylococcus, Fleming claimed to have discovered Penicillin on 3 September 1928.

Fleming said he returned to his laboratory after having spent August on holiday with his family. Before leaving, he had stacked all of his cultures of staphylococci on a bench in a corner of his laboratory. On returning, Fleming noticed that one culture was contaminated with a fungus, and that the colonies of staphylococci immediately surrounding the fungus had been destroyed, whereas other staphylococci colonies farther away were normal.

He did not discover the antibacterial property of the mould, but merely identified the optimum temperature required to grow the mould in the laboratory. We believed the story about the petri dish and moulds inhibiting growth, which we now know is not true. Spore from a laboratory one floor below, run by La Touche CJ, was transferred to Fleming's petri dish before the bacteria were added. At the time of the discovery, La Touche was working with the same mould found in Fleming's petri dish.

This marked the beginning of modern medicine, built on a foundation of lies and deceit, claiming to cure diseases and save lives. For years, scientists have published articles and books to rectify the error about the discovery of penicillin and other major advances in medicine, but the false story lives on.

HISTORY OF PENICILLIN

The discovery of penicillin is attributed to a Scottish scientist named Alexander Fleming. He showed that if Penicillium moulds were grown in the appropriate substrate, it would exude a substance with antibiotic properties. The development of penicillin for use as a medicine is attributed to the Australian pharmacologist Howard Walter Florey and the German chemist Ernst Chain. They were honored with the Nobel Prize for their discovery of the first antibiotic, "The Penicillin."

The contribution of a junior member of the team, biochemist Norman Heatly, possessed of a natural gift for ingenuity and invention, was virtually ignored. It was he who developed the technique of purifying and manufacturing of penicillin that has saved millions of lives. Heatley was assigned to work with Dr A J Moyer. They were able to push up yields of penicillin to 20 units per ml. Heatley stayed on in Peoria until December; then for the next six months he worked at Merck & Co, New Jersey.

When the result of their research was published, Moyer had omitted Heatley's name from the paper, despite an original contract which stipulated that any publications should be jointly authored.

Fifty years on we know that financial greed had led Dr Moyer to claim all the credit for himself. To acknowledge Heatley's part of the work would have made it difficult for Moyer to apply for patents as the sole inventor. In 1990 he was awarded the unusual distinction of an honorary Doctorate of Medicine from Oxford University, the first given to a non-medic in Oxford's 800-year history.

The most important discovery by Alexander Fleming about how bacteria develop resistance was ignored and cancelled. He warned doctors not to use penicillin unless there was a properly diagnosed reason for it to be used, and that if it were to be used, never to use too little or for too short a period of time. He said doctors must be "the custodians of antibiotics," to protect and not abuse this "Miracle Drug."

Unfortunately, members of our own profession ignored this warning and abused antibiotics, and so now, we have lost the one and only drug that actually cured infections and saved millions of lives.

INTRODUCTION

Management of common diseases as seen in primary and secondary medical care vary and depend on the primary care physician or nurse's experience of interpreting symptoms. Since 2003, the number of children less than five years, admitted in hospitals for less than twenty-four hours has doubled in the NHS (UK). These children were diagnosed to have serious URTI (upper respiratory tract infection), LRTI (lower respiratory tract infection and URTI (urinary tract infections) *(Peter Gill, Arch of Dis in Child, 2013).*

Presenting symptoms like runny nose, snuffles, or rhinitis have been diagnosed as common cold, and cough with fever as chest infection. Asthmatics were labeled as wheezy bronchitis, viral infections, sore throat, red ears and flu and often treated with antibiotics that you don't need. Western medicine is about diagnosing and eradication of infectious diseases using antibiotics and vaccinations. Unfortunately, we have failed to make our dream a reality, but successfully created a profession that has created micro-organisms that threaten our very existence. The more that we research these drugs, the more evidence we find that their benefits in most cases of minor illness are marginal; yet little evidence exists to support alternative treatments.

The duty of a primary care physician is to listen to the story of the illness, use his knowledge and experience to diagnose and offer advice to manage, not prescribe or promote drugs. We are not GOD who can save lives, but can help reduce pain, suffering, reduce or prevent complications and postpone death.

People in power (to reduce cost and increase profit), supported by some members of our profession have directly or indirectly forced doctors to offer healthcare based on algorithms and protocol. They claim this is based on evidence and so is in the interest of our profession. Doctors who felt their independence to manage patients has been systematically taken away, and protested saying this is not safe or is an unethical medical practice, have been criticized or ostracized.

"Common diseases commonly occur, rare diseases rarely happen." We neglected the so-called "Minor Ailments," managed with uncertainty often using common sense, and abused antibiotics. The Medical Research Council in 1997, funding for research into minor illness and the relict of self-limiting symptoms remains limited.

The doctor's first priority must be to satisfy himself or herself that there is no evidence of serious disease, and if so to reassure the patient accordingly. This may be all that is necessary; patients do not necessarily want advice on managing their illness, and traditional nursing advice (e.g., rest, copious fluids and regular paracetamol) is also not well supported by research.

When we started our research, we were surprised because there is not one study that supports or demonstrates why you must take antibiotics for 3, 5, 7, 10 or 14 days. The Center of Disease Control (CDC) and other institutions recommend completion of the course to help reduce the spread of resistant bacteria. It may not be necessary to prolong antibiotic treatment knowing bacterial infection can be cleared from our body after taking three doses. Prolonging treatment that may not be necessary may cause more harm to the environment and our body. Scientists have published articles to prove one dose of antibiotic will kill good germs in our body and we will be colonized with resistant bacteria for 6 to 8 weeks.

Low dose antibiotics, spirits, alcohol hand wash or antibiotic creams or drops kill harmless bacteria and help resistant bacteria flourish in our hands, eyes, skin or intestines.

The most important advice about bacteria developing resistance, by Alexander Fleming was ignored. He warned doctors "not to use penicillin unless there was a properly diagnosed reason for it to be used, and that if it were used, never to use too little, or for too short a period."

It is important for you to know, drugs must be taken once, twice, three or five times as advised because this is based on pharmacokinetics. Some drugs like antibiotics must reach optimum concentration (good peak) to help kill bacteria (bactericidal), if not the bacteria will stop multiplying (bacteriostatic) and develop resistance.

If you have bacterial infection and the antibiotic recommended is the right one, then you will start feeling better soon after you take the third dose. If the symptoms are not resolved and you are not feeling better, then the infection is likely to be caused by a virus or the bacteria which is resistant to the antibiotic. Please return to your doctors and ask for advice if you are not better after taking three doses.

Drugs used to treat diabetes, thyroid problem, mental illness, fits and other long-term problems must be maintained within a narrow range (optimum therapeutic level), if not they do not work, or are toxic if the dose is high.

Doctors must also be sensitive to the patient's beliefs and expectations, or 'agenda'. They may have attended in order to legitimize their illness to an employer, or at the insistence of a relative. Social factors, such as work, impending holiday or examination, will often be of far greater importance to patients than any medical issues, and will inevitably influence their assessment of the relative risks and benefits of any treatment.

In western medicine the 'placebo effect' is regarded as a nuisance, which interferes with the evaluation of the 'real' effects of a treatment in clinical trials. Yet the placebo effect is itself very real, and represents the influence of the patient's belief on the intrinsic healing ability of the body. You can harness this effect very easily, by being positive and emphasizing that a good recovery is likely. The placebo effect of any treatment that you suggest will be enhanced by the fact that you have recommended it, particularly. We have tested this hypothesis and know it is very essential for doctors to build good rapport and for patients to have access to their advice 24/7, 365 days to help us fight the threat to humanity, our profession and our lives.

If you have established good relations with the doctor, they must try to avoid destroying this effect by being too evidence based. Doctors must know it is unethical to offer treatment that is not required or withholding available treatment that helps patients. For example, prescribing simple linctus to suppress cough, statin, vitamin pills or tonics to help boost immunity – there's no evidence that this offers any benefit to the patient – must be discouraged. Yes, therapy (placebo effect) that makes the patient feel better is likely to accelerate the healing process, but doctors must know introducing drugs and chemicals into our body alter physiological process and so may be inflicting more harm than good.

Unfortunately, changes implemented in medical school training, over-enthusiastic urge to perform tests and investigations and giving less importance to clinical examinations has resulted in the loss of human face and made people not trust family physicians.

Discouraging patients from accessing healthcare is unethical because we know common symptoms are common but let us not forget serious illnesses are also present with symptoms that make you assume you have a minor ailment. By discouraging patients with the so-called "Minor Ailments" from consulting a doctor or visiting hospital and receiving the right treatment, we are inflicting pain and suffering and not preventing them from developing complications. Knowing that the cost of healthcare will increase to treat or manage complications because of hospitalization that can result in long-term problems, and even death, we must help bring in changes and defend our medical ethics.

MAYA is the only tool that is designed based on clinical acumen to help you differentiate minor illness from serious illness. We feel this simple tool will reduce access to doctors when you must not, and encourage you to consult if the collection of symptoms suggests the illness you suffer is potentially serious.

We sincerely hope, nurses, doctors and people like you will support, offer suggestion or recommend better alternatives if there are any, so that we can share our knowledge and experience and join hands to make sure our children as adults in the future are happy and healthy.

WHAT WE KNOW

Penicillin is the first drug that interfered with the protein synthesis of bacterial cell wall, but is useless against many other microbes such as fungi, virus, and bacteria like Mycoplasma, emerging infections and Gram-negative bacteria. These micro-organisms have membranes which prevent penicillin from penetrating them or the walls are not made of proteins. Some bacteria have changed their "genetic programs," which allows them to grab the antibiotic and spit it out.

These changes in the genetic programs can be in the form of chromosomal mutations, acquisition resistance genes, or through transposition pathogenicity. An example of a chromosomal mutation is the increasing number of cases of penicillin resistant Neisseria gonorrhoea. The bacteria spread occurs through "vertical evolution" (multiply) bacterial population growth but the most common method by which antibiotic resistance is acquired is through the conjugation called "horizontal evolution." This is much faster and makes different strains of micro-organisms resistant to drugs and chemicals we know.

In this method the bacteria need not multiply to spread their plasmid during conjugation. These plasmids often code for resistance to several antibiotics at once. The third method is transferring the genes that appear on the DNA and carry the codes that make the infection more successful. These transposable elements allow the genes to jump from bacteria to bacteria or simply from chromosome to plasmid within the organism.

Bacteria have evolved numerous methods, which simply destroy or limit the activity of the antibiotic. The beta-lactamases are enzymes, which render the penicillin-like antibiotics dysfunctional. Some bacteria can deactivate antibiotics by adding chemical groups to them by addition of a phosphate group. Other bacteria accomplish a similar effect by addition of an acetyl group.

Some bacteria acquire resistance by simply not allowing the antibiotic to enter the cell. The bacterium mentioned above, Neisseria gonorrhoea, has altered some proteins, thereby stopping uptake of the antibiotic. Some bacteria have intricate pumping mechanisms to expel the drug when it gains entry to their cell. Finally, bacteria may mutate the gene for the target macromolecule with which the antibiotic is supposed to bind. For example, tetracyclines binding by alterations in the ribosomal proteins that prevent tetracycline from binding but still allow the ribosome to function.

MECHANISM OF DEVELOPING RESISTANCE

Antimicrobial resistance occurs wherever antimicrobials are used in the community, on the farm, and in the hospital or long-term care facility. It is extremely important to understand the mechanisms by which micro-organisms can elude the effects of antimicrobial agents, as well as the factors that support and promote antimicrobial resistance. If conditions are right, a single bacterium can divide rapidly and produce a billion offspring in a single day.

Surviving microbes become dominant, adapting quickly to changing environmental conditions, including the introduction of new antimicrobial agents. Furthermore, multiple resistance mechanisms in a single bacterial pathogen are becoming the norm. This complicates treatment of these infections, increasing morbidity, mortality and healthcare costs.

TYPES OF RESISTANCE

Natural Resistance

It is the natural protection the organism has, such as the outer membrane of gram-negative bacteria, E. coli, resistance to vancomycin because vancomycin is too large to pass through the cell wall. All strains of a particular bacterial species will exhibit the same modes of resistance, and little can be done to change them.

Acquired Resistance

Does non-inherited change take place in the genetic composition of a microorganism so that an antibiotic that was once effective is no longer effective?

Specific mechanisms of acquired resistance that makes antibiotics ineffective:

Drug inactivation: Bacteria acquire gene-encoding enzymes that inactivate or destroy antimicrobial agents before they reach their bacteria.

Cell wall changes: The bacterial outer membrane becomes impermeable to the antibiotics.

Altered targets: The target site is altered by mutation of genes so that it evades the action of or no longer binds the antibiotics agent.

Efflux pump: The bacteria acquire an efflux pump that expels the antibiotics before it reaches its target within the cell.

Bypass targets: Mutations in bacterial DNA change the target enzyme in a metabolic pathway to bypass the primary target.

Inactivating enzymes: Are powerful facilitators of resistance used by many serious gram-negative microbes. These enzymes are capable of hydrolyzing wide range of antibiotics, including second and third-generation cephalosporins. Pathogens that produce these enzymes are difficult to treat and are increasingly responsible for serious healthcare-associated infections

In the presence of large dose of antibiotics, bacteria are killed or, if the dose is low, they stop multiplying and develop resistance. Almost every common bacteria we know carries resistance genes. They survive, reproduce and rapidly spread in our community. We hope you can understand the gravity of the problem we are in and help us reduce this spread so that scientists and doctors can find new methods to fight infections.

Unfortunately we were not fortunate to have developed a drug similar to antibiotics that kill viruses nor do we have enough knowledge about viruses. The Anti-viral drugs we have can only slow down the rate of multiplication and so reduce the number of people getting infected (viral shedding). They seldom cure viral infections and our body learns to protect us from subsequent infections. Scientists used this knowledge to help develop vaccination like Measles, Mumps and Rubella (MMR), flu and polio to prevent spreading infections.

This is a striking example of the evolutionary principle of natural selection. Initially, the resistant bacteria passed on their resistance genes to their offspring and subsequently other microbes like virus, fungus and parasites picked up the genes.

As we predicted in 2005, **"This is a war we may never win."** An army of twenty-two bacteria, numerous viruses, TB, Malaria and fungus armed with resistant genes, enzymes and lethal chemicals are likely to wipe out a generation in the next few years.

The only option we think we have is "MAYA" to help us identify infected people and isolate them as quickly as possible. Allowing people with infection to visit clinics, surgery and hospital will help these micro-organisms to infect other patients in the waiting room, healthcare workers and rapidly spread in the community killing thousands more.

TOP 10 DRUG-RESISTANT MICROORGANISMS		
Microorganisms	Examples of Diseases Caused	Drugs Resistant To
1. *E. coli* and other Enterobacteriaceae	Bacteremia, pneumonia, urinary tract and surgical wound infections	Aminoglycosides, beta-lactam antibiotics, chloramphenicol, trimethoprim
2. *Enterococcus*	Bacteremia, urinary tract and surgical wound infections	Aminoglycosides, beta-lactam antibiotics, erythromycin, vancomycin
3. *Haemophilus influenzae*	Epiglottitis, meningitis, otitis media, pneumonia, sinusitis	Beta-lactam antibiotics, chloramphenicol, tetracycline, trimethoprim
4. *M. tuberculosis*	Tuberculosis	Aminoglycosides, ethambutol, isoniazid, pyrazinamide, rifampin
5. *Neisseria gonorrhoeae*	Gonorrhea, pelvic inflammatory disease, urethritis	Beta-lactam antibiotics, spectinomycin, tetracycline
6. *P. falciparum* (protozoan)	Malaria	Chloroquine
7. *P. aeruginosa*	Bacteremia, pneumonia, urinary tract infections	Aminoglycosides, beta-lactam antibiotics, chloramphenicol, ciprofloxacin, tetracyclines, sulfonamides
8. *Shigella dysenteriae*	Severe diarrhea	Ampicillin, trimethoprim, sulfamethoxazole, chloramphenicol, tetracyclines
9. *S. aureus*	Bacteremia, endocarditis, pneumonia, skin surgical wounds, urinary infections	Chloramphenicol, ciprofloxacin, clindamycin, erythromycin, beta-lactam antibiotics, rifampin, tetracycline, trimethoprim
10. *S. pneumoniae*	Meningitis, otitis media, pneumonia	Aminoglycosides, chloramphenicol, erythromycin, penicillin

THREAT TO MEDICAL PROFESSION

"Resistance" is the capacity of an organism (human, animal or plant) to defend itself against other organisms, chemicals or environmental changes that threaten their existence. Bacteria, virus, fungus or parasites have been developing new methods to withstand the effects of a harmful chemical, physical or environmental agent for millions of years. The discovery of antibiotics and their widespread application in healthcare early in the 1940s was one that changed the way we lived and behaved.

Advances in medicine, no longer limited to diagnosing diseases, perform major surgical procedures, transplant organs, fertilize eggs in test-tubes to create embryos and claim to cure many diseases. The so-called "Miracle cures" highlighted by some members of our own profession made people live under an illusion that we can cure diseases and save lives.

In 1989, we realized this illusion has come to an end; the bacteria have started to fight back. They are stronger, armed with six enzymes, have passed on the technology and know-how to viruses and bacteria and have created an army of eighteen micro-organisms that can wipe out a generation in a few days. They have proved to be stronger, cleverer and have more advanced technology and know-how to manipulate their genetic vulnerability to drugs and chemicals kill them.

As antibiotics were increasingly used to treat illnesses in humans and animals the degree and complexity of antimicrobial resistance has grown. The genes of dead resistance bacteria provide a ready supply of mechanisms that allow other micro-organisms to swiftly develop resistance to new antibiotics.

Just like bacteria, viruses, parasites, and fungi have learned to survive and have become a major problem that is now considered one of the greatest threats to humanity.

Politicians, scientists and pharmaceutical companies are living under an illusion and using their network of media to make people believe we have the knowledge, technology and know-how to develop new antibiotics or drugs that can cure illness. Unfortunately, doctors are not in any position, nor have the technology to slow down the spread of infections.

We must first understand how bacteria, viruses and fungus are able to mount their clever defenses before we can contemplate treatment, management or cure. Using this knowledge of the genetics and mechanisms of resistance, scientists may discover new ways to fight infections.

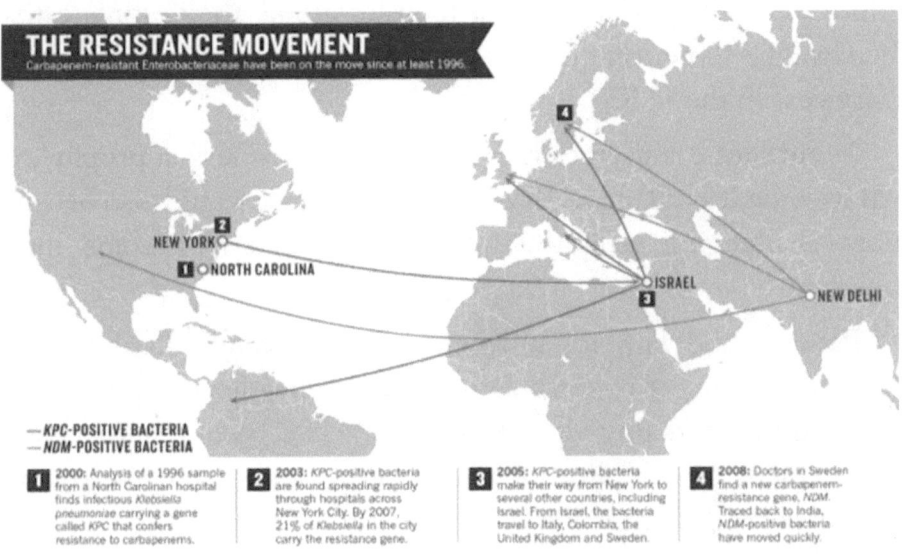

ANTIBIOTICS AND SURGERY

Infections and deaths of patients who need antibiotics in order to safely get through surgery and chemotherapy will increase. If antibiotic effectiveness drops by another 30 per cent from the current levels, that might result in an additional 120,000 infections for U.S. cancer and surgery patients and 6,300 infection-related deaths each year. A 70% decline in antibiotic effectiveness might lead to 280,000 more infections and 15,000 more deaths in USA.

Ten most common surgeries that involve prophylactic antibiotics are hip fracture surgery, pacemaker implantation, surgical abortion, spinal surgery, total hip replacement, caesarean section, transrectal prostate biopsy, appendectomy, abdominal hysterectomy and colorectal surgery. For prostate biopsies alone, they estimate that there will be 42 per cent of post-procedure infections – 13,320 cases, every year in the U.S.

As antibiotic resistance rates rise, it is inevitable that prophylaxis will become less effective. Treatment for cancer would also become more challenging as antibiotic resistant bacteria become more prevalent.

Patients and families must now start thinking hard because they will encounter two problems (1) Complications and death due to anesthesia and post-op infection. (2) The cost of surgery and management of complications is likely to double and there is no guarantee the patient will live.

In India, 97% of patients, USA 700,000 and Europe 400,000 are bankrupted after hospitalization. The escalating cost of managing the patients in hospitals will be devastating for families and children left behind after we die and so it is our duty to help bring in changes to reduce cost of healthcare.

Ten million people could die every year from 2050 onwards unless sweeping global changes are agreed to tackle increasing resistance to antibiotics, which can turn common illness into killers, a report

Commissioned by the British government. (Deccan Herald; 20/05/2016)

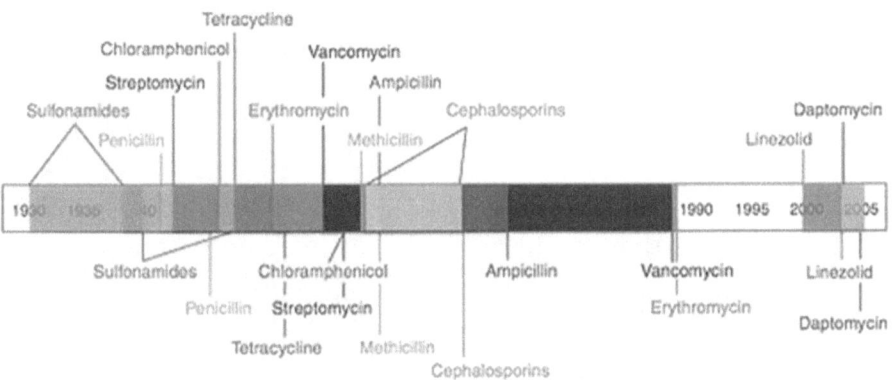

HOW TO AVOID ANTIBIOTIC ABUSE

Four Communication Strategies to help reduce antibiotic abuse were advised by CDC:

Provide a specific diagnosis to help patients feel validated. For example, say "viral bronchitis" instead of referring to an illness as "just a virus." Recommend symptomatic relief and share normal findings as you go through your examination.

Discuss potential side effects of antibiotic use, including adverse effects and resistance.

Inform patients that antibiotics are not as safe as we imagined and so are drugs that are harmful. Lastly, explain to the patient or parent what to expect over the next few days including that you will re-evaluate their situation and prescribe antibiotics if it becomes medically appropriate.

If you are on antibiotics prescribed by a doctor or nurse working in walk-in-clinic, in emergency care or out of hours service but not better after taking three doses, then please request your doctor to consult a microbiologist or refer you to hospital. Common infections caused by E.Coli, staphylococcus, streptococcus are now very difficult to treat. Changing and swapping antibiotics or advising you to continue treatment for 10 or 14 days can result in serious complications like septicemia and death.

Recent studies on some infections such as pneumonia and urinary tract infections suggest that shorter courses of treatment are just as effective, and less toxic, than longer courses. It is important for clinicians to be aware of evidence that can help guide the optimal duration of therapy. Some doctors blame patients who demand antibiotics when they aren't indicated, some will blame healthcare providers who are in a hurry to get patients out of the office, and others will blame the lack of rapid diagnostic tests to make prescribing decisions. There are numerous problems with many contributing factors and will require multifaceted solutions.

Recent study estimated ten (10) million deaths every year by 2050, if rapid tests to help diagnose an treat are not developed. Unfortunately, the media does not understand the gravity of the problem our profession is now facing. We have not been successful in understanding the tools or methods used to defend bacteria from antibiotics. Then how can we dream of inventing a "Miracle drug" that can kill an army of different bacteria, viruses and fungi. Since the 1980s we have not understood how MRSA (Methicillin Resistant Staph Aureus) operates, spreads and kills people, nor do we have a simple test to differentiate MSSA (Methicillin Sensitive Staph Aureus).

In the last two decades, nearly 70% of doctors requested tests, scans and performed procedures to boost their income. This has made people like you that tests and investigations are essential are essential to diagnose illness and so demand for investigations and antibiotics. We have spent our entire life diagnosing serious illnesses in acute and intensive care and were not fortunate to have tests or investigations to help us diagnose an illness in twenty minutes. We mastered the art of clinical examination, used our knowledge, experience and helped hundreds if not thousands of adults and children survive.

MAYA was developed with great passion to help us reduce the spread of infections in our community and to help us protect our children. Developing this tool has only brought us shame, made us suffer humiliation, inflicted pain and suffering on our family, isolated us from friends and made us suffer. We do not consider this the only solution, but we believe this is the only way forward knowing the situation we are in.

Allowing bacteria to infect more people and multiply can only make the invaders stronger and more virulent and resistant. Our mission is to share the secret and educate you to think like we did and help you learn more about symptoms and signs to differentiate minor from serious illnesses. You will learn how doctors all over the world use a combination of a few symptoms to derive at "Clinical Diagnosis," perform tests and investigations to confirm or diagnose illnesses and offer advice or treatment.

More information about appropriate antibiotic use and tools, including a symptomatic prescription pad can be found on CDC's Website. Also read more about antibiotics, recommended dose, duration of treatment, side effects and any information about resistance and sensitivity.

MANAGEMENT OF MINOR ILLNESS

In the past twenty years, we have seen that the standard of care in primary care has declined. Year on year, there has been a sharp rise in costs, litigations, medical errors, hospitalizations and death rate. People in power, institutions and the Royal Colleges are not coming forward to accept the fault and are strongly advocating "Evidence based practice."

In 1996, we published a letter in a medical journal and criticized authors supporting changes in medical school education and training of doctors in hospitals. In 1999, we stopped working as doctors in the hospital because we could not ignore the pain and suffering inflicted due to medical errors committed by doctors who followed guidelines and protocols. It was very obvious; the newly qualified doctors were made to give more importance to this so-called Evidence Based Medicine (EBM), ignoring consultation and clinical skills to derive at a diagnosis and offer advice or treatment.

The reason why we are failing in healthcare is because the name "Evidence" is deceiving people and some doctors. Not many healthcare professionals understand how to interpret the result and advice treatment. EVB does not quantify any treatment but merely suggests possible causes of some illness.

As a clinician, we cannot accept "Treatment suggested in EBM is 100% correct." In 1980s, we were collecting information (audit) to help us identify our mistakes and rectify. Evidence Based Medicine was developed based on the data we collected. To tell you frankly, we would have given you a robot called "MAYA" if the data we collected had helped us derive at a diagnosis for illness and offer treatment.

Evidence based medicine merely provides information like "Streptococcus is the commonest organism identified in 80% of throat swabs taken in patients diagnosed as tonsillitis," "Staphylococcus aureus is colonized in the nose of 30% of people" or "70% patients have better control of epilepsy if treated with drug A when compared with Drug B." This does not mean to say we can give diagnosis or offer treatment based on the information.

The doctors who did not accept and criticized this algorithmic or protocol based approach to offer treatment were harassed, humiliated and ostracized by members of our own profession. Doctors who accept this algorithmic approach are safe but we know you and I are not safe. If you happen to be one of the people in the 20% growing some bacteria in your throat, other than Streptococcus and are treated with penicillin as recommended in the protocol, you will soon develop "Septicemia" and die. 37,000 people are said to develop septicemia and die every year in UK since 2006. This is one fact we have never heard or seen before 2006.

Prescribing antibiotics to patients diagnosed as URTI (upper respiratory tract infection), LRTI (lower respiratory tract infections), UTI (urinary tract infection), chest infection, flu or viral infections must stop. Prescribing one broad-spectrum antibiotic to infection labeled as URTI is not only expensive but also harmful to patients. Doctors or nurses must localize infection like tonsillitis, otitis media (not ear infection), rhinitis (not runny nose), sinusitis, and pharyngitis and use the right antibiotic because the colony of bacteria in throat is not the same one that lives in sinus or ear.

Where differences are apparent, doctors should access up-to-date information and be vigilant about emerging bacteria and viruses. High-quality research evidence, CDC publications to aid discussion and help doctors manage infection changes every week if not every day. Critical analysis of published research has become highly complex and very time-consuming; thankfully there are now several agencies such as the Cochrane Collaboration, which analyze the evidence on your behalf, and provide easy access to this information on the Internet.

This is our contribution to help educate you about common illnesses that can be managed by you and do not require help from doctors, nurses or chemist. We are sharing information about wrong doings and mistakes that have cost lives or made people suffer. Please use this book as reference and double check information in medical textbooks. Some of the information shared on the is also not reliable and so can cause harm to your family, friends or you.

We hope to create a network of doctors and patients from all over the world, ease communication, and share information and knowledge to help us **"Bring Tears of Happiness,"** and fight infections for a healthier and happier tomorrow.

ABOUT US

The discovery of penicillin marks a true turning point in the history of medicine and humanity. We were fortunate to work, gain knowledge, perform procedures, and learn how to manage complicated medical illnesses as taught by the very doctors who are the architects of modern medicine and surgery.

We have shared our knowledge, experiences, and skills with our students hoping they will bring tears of happiness in the eyes of people who trust our profession.

We have spent the last decade trying to understand how and why we allowed some members of our profession to commercialize these skills and knowledge that were bestowed upon us by our teachers to help alleviate pain and suffering in the universe.

As physicians, we felt very uncomfortable because we have lost the clinical independence in deciding upon the care of a person for whom we are medically responsible.

The World Medical Association Declaration states that a doctor must have clinical independence in deciding upon the care of a person for whom he or she is medically responsible. The physician's fundamental role is to alleviate the distress of his or her fellow human beings, and no motive, whether personal, collective or political, shall prevail against this higher purpose.

We were naïve to believe that the people in powerful institutions, associations, organizations, and our fellow physicians would support the physician and his or her family in the face of threats or reprisals for defending medical ethics.

Knowing that micro-organisms threaten our very existence, we are striving to share our experience, knowledge and information, and to help you acquire the skill required to reduce wasted consultations, cross infections and abuse of antibiotics.

INTRODUCTION TO MAYA

Humanity is now facing a mortal enemy that surpasses our own Intelligence. A tiny microorganism that has indeed, brought us to our knees… It has learned from us, adapted to us, and now exploits our genetic vulnerability, with lethal precision. As the death toll mounts, our greed, over-enthusiastic urge to encourage consultation, perform tests, procedures, hospitalization and addiction to antibiotics escalates at alarming rates.

Pharmaceuticals companies, medical device manufacturers, government and even some doctors reject this threat labeled as "The Ticking Time Bomb." A deadly epidemic that could have global implications is quietly sweeping India. Infants are born with bacterial infections that are resistant to most known antibiotics, and more than 58,000 died last year as a result, a recent study found.

MAYA is a tool developed to help reduce the cultural dependency of doctors to help diagnose illness and offer treatment. Using MAYA we can reduce delay in diagnosis, medical errors, cross infections and cost of providing basic health care advice and management of illness.

The experiences of patients with symptoms of physical or mental illnesses are so common they do not even pay much attention to what goes on in hospitals and clinics all over the world. When the doctors they consult request a number of tests to be done even for a common symptom, or insist on doing pathological tests, patients are pleased and often praise the doctors for taking care of them.

Though there is always suspicion of commission or perks for the doctor from such references, there is hardly anything that one can prove. Consultation with a doctor is confidential and so patients with a common symptom can be managed based on the doctor's mood, assessment of patients' financial status, emotional instability and expectations.

The benefits from offering special services purchasing drugs, vaccinations and equipment., to establishing diagnostic centers, offering triage service, training and education, help create jobs. Establishing colleges, nursing schools, hospitals and institutions like Royal Colleges, Medical Councils and Medical Associations that publish books and medical journals, and organize conferences, benefits a large number of doctors and politicians across the world.

Based on our personal experiences, we are now for the first time sharing the information about wrong doings and corruption in health care system that has brought us harm. This is not about control, return on investment, blaming and shaming but about honest effort to help systemize healthcare.

We have now spent more than ten years studying the trend and know our contribution can only make a small dent in healthcare system. We are happy that this dent will bring in significant changes in fighting infections and saving lives.

WHY TRUST MAYA?

Our aim is to share our knowledge and experience, so that you are not helping the bacteria and viruses spread in our community killing our friends and our children. We provide you with the relevant information about common symptoms and diseases and teach you how we use the combination of three symptoms to differentiate minor from serious illnesses. This is what we taught our students and colleagues working as junior doctors for thirty years.

Visiting hospitals and health centres is now not as safe as it used to be, because hospitals, clinics and healthcare centers are not only colonized with bacteria that we cannot kill, but also with emerging infections. The fear of catching infection is also making patients with serious illnesses take self-medication, consult nurses or chemist to avoid consulting a doctor. The delay in access is making it more difficult for doctors to help because you can develop serious complications.

Please do not use our tool to offer advice or suggest treatment to friends and acquaintances. As doctors we know, some patients are not completely honest and do not share all the information they must. Offering advice to friends is not safe because they are likely to conceal information and so you may give them false reassurance resulting in delay, complications and death. Doctors, nurses, teachers and receptionists working in healthcare will find our MAYA will help reduce demand and organize their appointment system and help reduce waiting time.

Healthcare is all about trust and care. This App and tool was developed with a passion to protect you from complications that occur due to wrong diagnosis and delay in treatment. We have taken meticulous care, tested this hypothesis for almost six years and found it to be safe. We have deliberately removed some symptoms that require clinical examination by an experienced doctor. We will share our knowledge and experience and offer you the correct information about common symptoms to educate you. If you find the information we provide and share is not right or misleading, please share the information to help us bring tears of joy in this world of sorrow, discomfort and uncertainty.

The information available in medical literatures and published on the internet can often make you anxious resulting in wasted consultations. We sincerely hope our work will help your family and you reduce cost, travel and complications. In return we expect you to REGISTER and **NOT HOLD US LIABLE** for harm (physical, psychological or financial) that you think may have occurred directly or indirectly after using our tools.

"Scientists were so pre-occupied with whether or not they could, they did not stop to think if they should…"-- Jurassic Park. It's ironic, a fantasy movie, which aptly describes the medical crisis we face today, I am talking about Ebola, and antibiotic resistant bacterial infections.

We are now facing a mortal enemy that surpasses our own Intelligence. A tiny microorganism that has indeed, brought us to our knees.

WHY USE MAYA?

Pharmaceuticals, medical device manufacturers, government and even some doctors reject this, "Elephant in the doctors room." By not guarding the miracle drug as custodians, we allowed antibiotics to fatten chickens and treat animals, encouraged nurses to use our clinical skill to diagnose illness and prescribe drugs, and chemists to sell antibiotics without prescription.

Sadly, they who dared to speak up, were ridiculed, ignored, dismissed and often ostracized, by institutions and members of our own profession. Yet the death toll mounts, while our greed, addiction towards and over-enthusiastic urge to encourage consultations, perform tests and procedures, hospitalization and antibiotic abuse escalate at alarming rates.

We have now lost the one and only drug that helped us fight infections, learn more about our body, make advances in medicine possible, perform surgical procedures, transplant surgery, IVF and save millions of people.

Common diseases commonly occur, rare diseases rarely happen but we neglected these so-called "Minor Ailments." Symptoms of common disease are under-researched, little understood and managed with uncertainty and often using common sense.

Some symptoms make patients anxious and so they access information via Internet or books. This often results in increasing anxiety, demanding emergency appointments in surgery or visiting hospital. The culture of dependency on doctors has increased cost resulting in patients consulting friends, nurses and chemist resulting in delay, complications and death.

Presenting symptoms like runny nose, snuffles, or rhinitis have been diagnosed as common cold and cough as chest infection. Asthmatics were labeled as wheezy bronchitis, tendency, viral infections, and flu and often treated with antibiotics.

Similarly, doctors also encouraged patients with high fever, sore throat, and earache to access healthcare professionals. Now it is mandatory not to prescribe antibiotics for "Minor Ailments."

Views on the common diseases as seen in primary and secondary medical care vary and depend on the primary care physician or nurse's experience of interpreting symptoms.

Some patients exaggerate their symptoms, pain, demand tests or treatment but others who trust their doctors conceal their emotions and receive the best advice or treatment.

Offering advice or treatment based on algorithms and protocol is unethical because this can often results in errors and delay in diagnosis that may result in long-term complications. Doctors must be allowed to use their knowledge and skill to diagnose disease and offer treatment only if necessary.

We have developed a simple solution, which was tested by some patients and found to be safe. Our mission is not reducing the cost of providing the best healthcare service, but helping and educating you to "Alleviate Your Pain and Suffering," and reduce complications in patients who trust members of our profession. To protect fellow humans from unethical medical practices that may cause harm.

In the past we could diagnose various infections based on some symptoms and name the disease. Now the bacteria are different because they have developed resistance to various antibiotics.

Allowing non-medically trained persons like chemists, nurses, assistants or friends to diagnose and prescribe antibiotics without proper training and supervision is an unethical medical practice.

New research has revealed how healthcare providers have become the victims of a demand-led culture.

In countries like UK, emergency care is now so bad that nurses are treating thousands of patients instead of doctors, because they are cheaper to employ.

Please download Dr MAYA App, Register and request your family doctor to download MAYA Dr and join our effort to create a local group and be prepared. Always use Dr MAYA before you visit hospital or consult a doctor. This will help you reduce delay, cost, cross infections and antibiotic abuse.

HOW CAN MAYA HELP?

We have seen patients developing minor and serious complications because they did not consult a doctor early, due to fear of cost, cross infections or received false reassurance from nurse or chemist.

As doctors working in acute and intensive care for almost thirty years, we have used this simple tool to priorities consultation, treatment or hospitalization.

MAYA thinks like a doctor working in a hospital or Emergency Care. She presents you a list of common symptoms and allows you to choose the answer to a few leading questions.

Based on your response, MAYA will grade the severity of your illness. Once she decides you may require clinical examination, tests or investigations, she will advise you to speak to or consult a doctor.

If the symptom cannot be managed at home or in primary care, she will advise you to go to hospital as an emergency.

MAYA is the only tool developed with passion to help you reduce wasted consultation, cost, medical errors, cross infections, hospitalization and antibiotic abuse…

"Tell me and I will forget. Teach me and I will remember. Involve me and I will learn."

— Benjamin Franklin

"Knowledge of Health Is Knowledge of Life" and the way to make healthcare affordable is by educating you and letting you be involved in the decision making process. This symptom checker tool is based on "Clinical Acumen" (How doctors think) and not based on the

"Manchester Triage Scoring System" developed by nurses and medical students.

Knowledge and understanding about health and well-being has advanced, but access to healthcare professionals has not seen a similar improvement. It's sad to hear that forty five million Americans are not insured, in UK the access to doctors has become very difficult as well as expensive, and in India, 97% of patients accessing healthcare are bankrupted.

Seventy percent of the cost of providing healthcare is spent on medical professionals (doctors). To save cost some healthcare providers in some countries are allowing nurses and non-medically trained personnel to diagnose and treat patients. We identified minor and major complications that have, as a result of this less than optimal approach to diagnosis, resulted in pain and suffering to people just like you.

Our mission is to help you learn more about your symptoms and reduce short and long-term complications or death. Arriving at medical diagnosis and deciding on appropriate treatment based on algorithms, protocols and/or guidelines is not safe. This is unethical too because it often leads to a delay in treatment.

MINOR ILLNESS

It has not been easy for doctors to differentiate minor from serious illness. Since 2006 nurses working in the NHS (UK) with no formal medical school training are clinically examining, diagnosing, advising and prescribing treatment. The result of this callous attitude is very evident. We have meticulously collected data and identified combinations of symptoms that can be safely managed by nurse or chemist. If you are not happy or you do not have nurse-led practice, walk-in-clinic or nurse triage service, please speak to a doctor

MODERATE ILLNESS

Must be seen by a Doctor who may clinically examine, perform tests or do investigation. Patients with the combination of some symptoms must not be examined, advised or treated by people who have not received formal medical school training. Delay in diagnosis and treatment may result in minor or serious complication or even death.

SERIOUS ILLNESS

Must be treated as an Emergency by a specialist in a hospital and not managed at home by family doctors, nurses or chemist.

© 2003 KMS Patent Protected GB1004457.6 All rights Reserved

ILLNESS OR ILLUSION?

Since Antibiotics became widely available, patients have been encouraged to consult and seek advice early, the result of which was often the prescription of a course of antibiotics. This has not only undermined your confidence as a patient, but also made bacteria stronger and more resistant to antibiotic agents.

Doctors have stopped managing illness based on history and clinical examinations and give more importance to tests and investigation. Unfortunately, this over-enthusiastic urge to encourage consultation, investigations and performing tests has made us lose the human face of medicine and increased the cost.

When patients describe the symptoms for which they are seeking professional attention, they are also reporting the story of an illness as they have lived, and remembered it.

(Srivatsa KM. QHJ (BMJ), 1996)

A working mother with a sick child needs an urgent help. Does this strike a chord?

What does she do? Rush to consult a family doctor, go to hospital and wait for hours in the out patient department or trauma centre in a local hospital.

According to World Medical Association Declaration, "A physician must have complete clinical independence in deciding upon the care of a person for whom he or she is medically responsible. The physician's fundamental role is to alleviate the distress of his or her fellow human beings, and no motive, whether personal, collective or political, shall prevail against this higher purpose."

Unfortunately, doctors do not have the clinical independence to stop unethical or sub-standard medical practice offered by healthcare providers. More administrators, more bureaucracy, tight budgets, over-enthusiastic urge to investigate, perform tests and hospitalization and abusing antibiotics are not the stuff of great healthcare provision.

After several years planning and research, we compiled a list of common symptoms that make people anxious to consult doctors.

We found, more than 70% of patients consulting a doctor as an emergency, did not have any serious illness that required clinical examination, tests or referral to a specialist in hospital. Using our findings, we created MAYA to help you learn how to differentiate:

FACTS ABOUT ANTIBIOTIC RESISTANCE

We can forgive you as a lay person for not knowing exactly what scientists mean by antibiotic resistance, but not if you are a doctor or a nurse. After reading numerous articles published in tabloid newspapers, we know very few people working in healthcare profession understand what's going on. What it means is bacteria becoming resistant or immune to the drugs we managed to kill and cure infections.

A new study published by Welcome Trust reported that almost no one really understands the problem or how serious it is. Even after Center of Disease Control (CDC) of The World Health Organization suggests that we're approaching a "post-antibiotic era," the end of modern medicine, not many doctors have stopped or reduced prescribing antibiotics.

Naming this as "Superbugs" and publishing articles, pictures and films to educate, pharmaceutical companies, equipment manufacturers, doctors and people are not giving much importance to this threat to humanity. Unless we take drastic steps and act very quickly, it could mean the end of modern medicine and billions will be wiped off this planet very soon.

People often talk to us about raising funds for cancer research, but not many help charities that are fighting antibiotic resistant bacterial infection, because they are not aware that chemotherapy and radiotherapy (the most common treatments for cancers) damage our body's own defenses against infection resulting in death.

Surgeons have used antibiotics saying it is necessary to prevent post-op infections. As antibiotics become unusable and sterilization techniques are failing to sterilize equipment and instruments, it will become impossible to prevent patients from getting infections. Eventually, everyday procedures such as appendectomies, hip replacements, and knee repairs – let alone open heart surgery – will be too dangerous to carry out.

We feel sad to say, the surgeons who behaved bad and did not acknowledge or share the reward with their microbiologists, virologists, immunologists and even physicians, will soon find it hard to continue to offer their services. This will bring an end to life-saving transplants, minimally invasive surgery and IVF.

Despite knowing the lives of post-operative patients are threatened with resistant bacterial infections, heart, lung, liver, and kidney and even face and womb transplants – are increasingly common. Drugs used to suppress rejection of transplanted organs (suppress their immune systems) and lack of antibiotics makes performing procedures unethical as this "can inflict pain and suffering."

Twenty-five to thirty percent of births in the UK are by caesarean section. This procedure is often done because the life of the mother or baby is at risk if allowed to give birth naturally. Majority of mothers get infections afterwards. The post-operative infection rate is not well known, but estimated to be 3% to 5%, that's about 4,000 women per year in Britain.

In the past majority of bacteria were picked up outside hospitals, but now most drug-resistant bacteria are caused by resistant bacteria colonized in hospitals. This rapid change will result in complications, long-term problems and even death in five or ten years.

Developing resistance is a perfect example of evolution in action. Antibiotics will kill almost all the bacteria it targets but the ones that survive are resistant to treatment. They reproduce every 15 to 20 minutes and so the next generation of bacteria will be colonized in your body in hours and infect your family and children.

In the 1970s, the first drug-resistant strain of gonorrhoea appeared and now we are only a few years away from gonorrhoea being completely untreatable. Doctors working in cancer hospitals are already struggling to treat infections in immunosuppressed cancer or transplant patients.

Outbreak of highly drug-resistant "super-gonorrhea" is sweeping across Britain and could become untreatable. Public Health England last September after the rare strain of the sexually transmitted superbug was detected in 34 people.

Failure to respond appropriately will jeopardies our ability to treat gonorrhea effectively and will lead to poorer health outcomes for individuals and society as a whole"

PHE said an increase in cases of super-gonorrhea was a "further sign of the very real threat of antibiotic resistance to our ability to treat infections".

The British Association for Sexual Health and HIV issued an alert to clinicians urging them to follow up cases of high-level drug resistant gonorrhea and trace their sexual partners. The spread of high-level azithromycin-resistant gonorrhea is a huge concern and it is essential that every effort is made to contain further spread.

Patients demand antibiotics from their doctors when they don't need them. Yes, it is difficult for patients or doctors to be 100% sure, but when the doctor say "No antibiotics," patients often complain saying the doctor is rude, or take legal action if post viral secondary bacterial infection occurs. Knowing that viral infection suppresses immunity, the doctor who acted in the interest of the patient is prosecuted and so not many doctors will refuse to prescribe.

Even after we spend time and explain viruses (are like elephant) are different from bacteria (are like ants), and antibiotics (are like match stick) can only kill bacteria because we do not have anti-viral drugs (like a double barrel gun) to kill virus (elephant), people have turned around and demanded antibiotics. You must know that taking antibiotics for your cold won't make you better, but it will make any bacteria that are in your system (and there are always trillions) develop resistance and so you can be a carrier who infects at home and in the community.

Doctors and institutions blame that the developing nations are abusing antibiotics because they are sold in shops without prescription. Yes, we agree it is wrong, but the number of people abusing is comparatively less than in the west. Globally, more people are dying from lack of access to basic antibiotics than from resistant ones. Most people think that it's the patient, not the bacterium inside the patient, that's becoming resistant, but the opposite is true.

So-called experts are advising you to take antibiotics for 5, 7, 10 or 14 days. We were unable to find any study that compares 5, 7, 10 or 14 days' course and prove it is necessary. Only study we could identify is one comparing short 3 days course to others. Theoretically we need 3 doses (good peak) to kill bacteria and may be 2–3 days will be sufficient to clear all infections. If the duration of treatment is prolonged, more antibiotics will be excreted in urine and stools and so pollute soil and water.

More than 50% of antibiotics worldwide are used on animals – "if one cow looks sick, they dose the whole herd," " Ponds full of the cattle treated with antibiotics are passing excrement that pollute water with antibiotic" – breeding grounds for resistant bacteria. These bacteria can easily jump from animals to cause diseases in humans.

It's not easy to find new antibiotics. Even if we find one now, it will take 20–40 years for us to manufacture and market it. The first antibiotic, penicillin, was discovered in 1800 but developed some 60 years later and this will never happen again.

We need new methods to control the spread of infections and not waste time trying to find a drug to kill bacteria or virus. A new antibiotic can cost literally billions to get to market and the pharmaceutical companies are not investing on drugs that are used for a week knowing bacteria will also develop resistance.

Once bacteria become resistant to an antibiotic, it might be decades before it can be used again. There has always been one glimmer of hope, as some scientists believe non-resistant bacteria may reproduce faster and eventually squeeze the resistant ones out if we stop using antibiotics.

We have been publishing articles, sharing information with various device manufacturers and institutions since 1989. The number of people talking about and recommending treatment method to control spread has been increasing day by day but the changes we expect have not. We hope our contribution to help you will bring in changes that will not only help you but also your family.

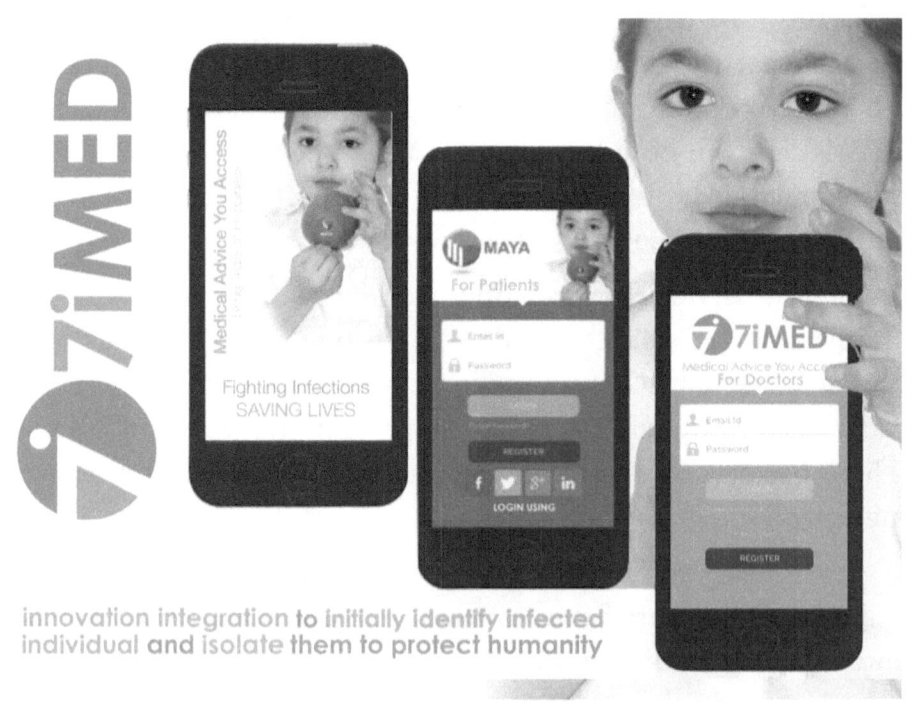

innovation integration to initially identify infected individual and isolate them to protect humanity

DR MAYA & MAYA DR APPS

Created by integrating MAYA with communication technology and information technology to help encourage members of our profession to share knowledge, innovate and develop products and methods to fight infection here and abroad.

Using advances in technology we have developed a system and a monitor to identify infected people (in hospitals, community, and country) initially, and help isolate them to protect humanity, as we know that we will not be able to develop or discover eighteen antibiotics to fight as many bacteria. I have just returned depressed from a conference in London because the pharmaceutical companies, scientists and microbiologists have no new antibiotics to offer and have also accepted it will not be possible to fight the threat of bacterial infection.

India is said to be a major threat to the world because the bacteria and TB are rapidly spreading in soil, water and sewage systems.

We offer a simple cost effective solution to help department of health to implement and monitor, so that we can avert an epidemic and not struggle to cope after hundreds or thousands of people die.

We begged members of my profession to shun their ego, share knowledge and information, communicate, and join hands with us to help us stop this "Elephant In The Room" that is now threatening our profession and our very existence

MEDICAL ADVICE YOU ACCESS

MAYA (Medical Advice You Access) was created initially to help receptionists and nurses working in nurse-led clinics, walk-in-clinics and emergency out of hours services to differentiate well from unwell patients and then refer unwell patients to doctors or hospital, if required.

By integrating our invention with IT, we have created the "FIRST TOOL TO HELP MONITOR INFECTIONS"

Doctors who download our Apps Maya Dr and register will help us create a network of doctors and patients. Once the doctor has downloaded, installed and registered on the system, his or her name will appear in the list of local doctors. Patients living in an area can choose their own local doctor or register with a different doctor.

Patients will be able to get information provided by that doctor, communicate 24/7, 365 days, send/receive letters or prescriptions and also book appointments. MAYA Dr can be linked to hospitals management system or we can offer help to digitalize and systemize healthcare in hospitals, clinics and Department of health.

Doctors can also offer video consultation, share notes via email and text message and also send prescriptions via email. Doctors can forward referral letters, sick notes and also search for information using the Internet while speaking to a patient.

This app will help doctors to prevent the spread of dangerously contagious diseases among patients. Patients with infections such as chicken pox, the MRSA infections, flu, Ebola and other emerging infections, can quickly be identified and the patients advised to visit health centers or hospitals thus helping to stop epidemics and pandemics in the future.

Registered Doctor can list symptoms, add information, videos, pictures and also personal video messages that patients can watch. Doctors can create a database in their own language; add telephone number of pharmacies, emergency services and other doctors working in hospitals or Health Centers in their area.

Doctors must advise your patients to download Dr MAYA, register, log in and choose you as their doctor. Once they are registered, they will be able to enter three symptoms, get your advice and communicate with you as required.

This is a simple tool created by a doctor with the passion to help other doctors offer their services to protect their fellow human beings and alleviate pain and suffering all over the world. Soon 7i will offer an opportunity for doctors to be listed as specialist private doctors who will offer telephone consultation for a nominal fee.

Department of Health, Hospitals, Airlines, Healthcare Service providers, embassies and doctors can create their own portal and offer services to registered users. This tool will reduce the number of receptionists, booking clerks, nurses and even junior doctors (Casualty Medical Officers).

Delay in registration, waiting in hospitals and clinics, medical errors and cost of providing care 24/7, 365 days will be reduced by 2/3. The most important benefit is to avoid infected patients entering Trauma or Accident centers resulting in death of staff and patients in waiting.

7i Med Ltd. offer the integrated innovation that is Dr MAYA, initially to help identify infected patients and isolate them to protect healthcare workers and thus humanity in general.

HOW DOES IT WORK?

We expect doctors, specialists, hospitals, companies, universities and institutions, government healthcare providers, medical colleges and education departments to download our Dr MAYA and create their own databases. Foreign nationals, diplomats and other visitors living in London or the UK will be able to get healthcare advice from doctors based in their own country. The NHS would no longer have to claim that they are losing money because of treating immigrants and other foreign nationals.

Patients download Dr MAYA and then add the name of a local doctor with that doctor's email and telephone number. Once our server receives the contact details of the new doctor, they will receive a confirmation notification. If a patient logs in and their symptoms suggest a serious, contagious, infection, that patient can be quickly isolated and their doctor informed.

Doctors can use Dr MAYA to add symptoms, change the ranking color of symptoms, insert video, pictures and also create an information sheet which patients can download. Doctors will advise patients to download Dr MAYA and ask them to choose him/her as their doctor. The patient will then be linked to their own doctors 24/7, 365 days.

Before booking an appointment the patient will log on and enter their symptoms. This is similar to calling a medical receptionist to explain why they need an appointment. Dr MAYA evaluates the symptoms and advises the patient based on knowledge and experience. It does not give an ad hoc answer like many receptionists will, but will give an answer based on the doctor's intelligence.

Patients will not be able to call a doctor if the Dr MAYA system has suggested the patient should go to a pharmacist or nurse or directly to a hospital. This reduces time-wasting consultations for non-threatening reasons like "I have a fever," head ache or wart, etc.

Dr MAYA will also stop patients abusing healthcare staff because of misdiagnoses or other problems: Dr MAYA's recommendations are always more accurate and related directly to the patient's problems.

Only patients who require clinical examination or specific tests will be advised to book an appointment. This will reduce emergency appointments by 80% because doctors will only see patients requiring face-to-face consultations.

Patients will be advised to call the 999 numbers if their symptoms are very serious. If their symptoms indicate a less threatening illness the patient will be advised to call the NHS 111 number. This will reduce the number of people dying because they have called 111 when they should have called 999.

The features 7i have provided are simple and provide clear options for both doctors and patients. Dr MAYA provides a common sense, practical solution to a major threat to humanity. Using Maya Dr and Dr MAYA will stop medical staff in isolation units from dressing up like an astronaut!

The Health Secretaries and Departments of Health in every country need seriously to think about the care they provide. If a country does not offer basic healthcare to people, Dr MAYA can. We must act now to prevent and control an uncontrollable tsunami of bacteria and viruses that could wipe out a generation.

7i think this is the only method we can use until scientists and pharmaceutical companies develop a new miracle cure to fight infections in the future.

The only immediately available alternate to treatment is the Maya system. Millions if not Billions will die if we continue to ignore this threat to humanity until scientists and pharmaceutical companies develop a one new antibiotic or think of alternate methods.

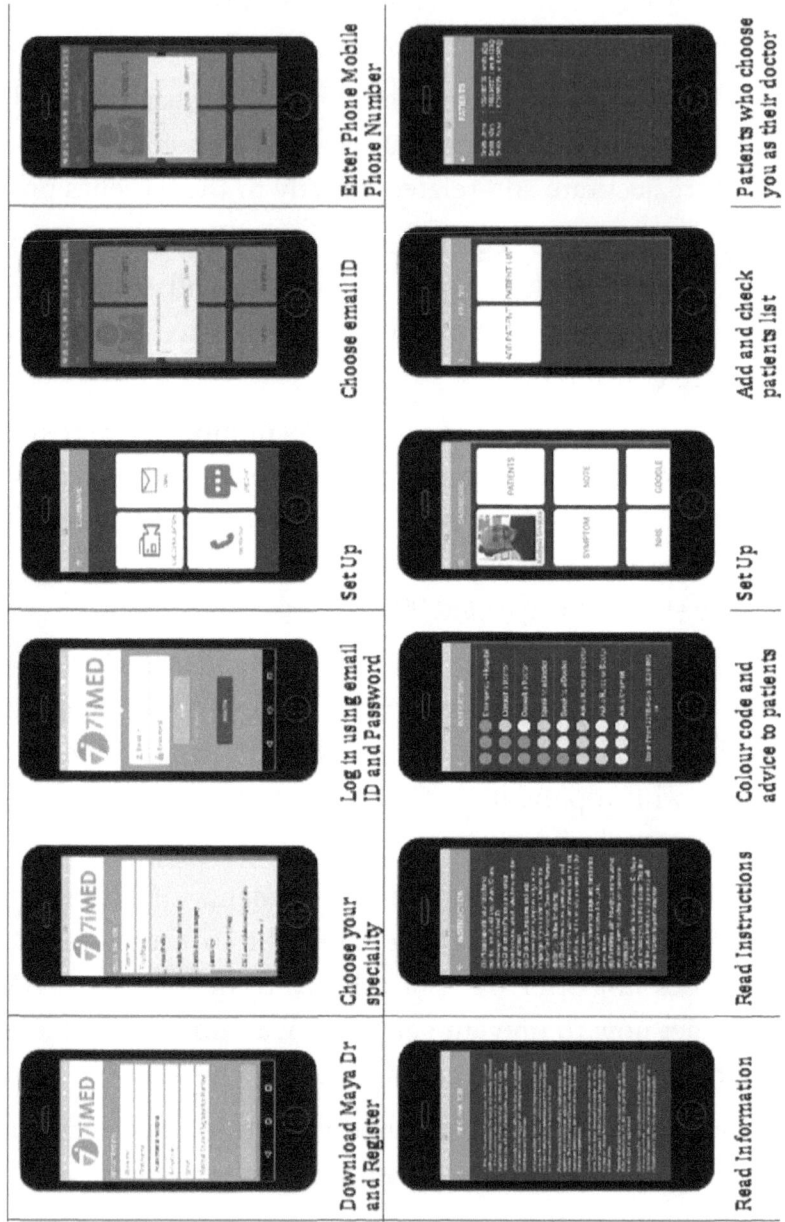

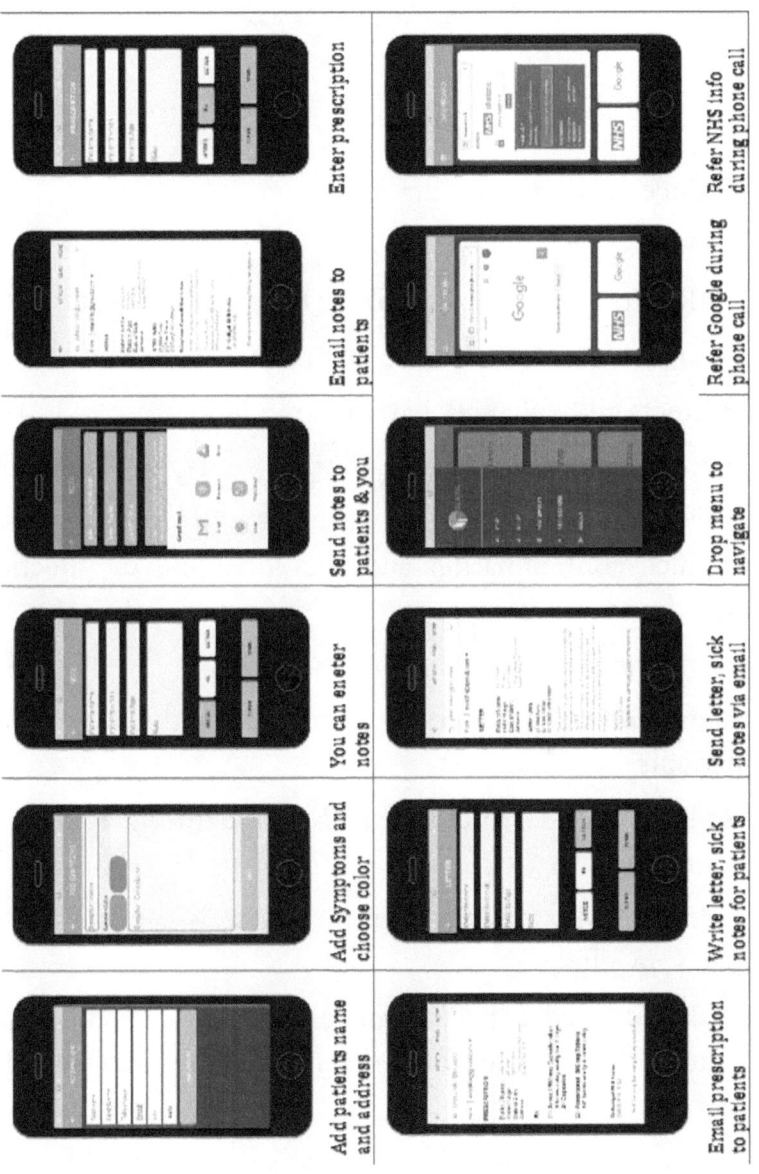

ADVANTAGES FOR HEALTH CARE PROVIDERS

- Reduce needless consultations
- Reduce staffing costs
- Reduce the number of booking clerks and receptionists
- Reduction of Primary care doctors and CMOs
- Protects and enhances patient confidentiality
- Patients easily diverted to another center or doctor if crisis occurs
- Reduce contamination and the spreading of infections in health centers
- Reduce antibiotic misuse and cost
- Reduction in epidemics by identifying and isolating infected patients
- Reduction of death of staff and people during epidemics and pandemics
- Identify and quarantine private hospitals because Dr MAYA picks up clusters
- Reduced need for Ambulance service as MAYA will only request Ambulance for serious conditions and not for false alarms
- Reduction of 60%-80% of patients accessing A&E
- Make doctors work efficiently and systemize healthcare advice

ADVANTAGE TO DOCTORS

- Able to offer 24/7, 365 day effective service
- Patients given effective and accurate treatment directly relating to the seriousness of their problem
- Patients will not be able to call if Dr MAYA has suggested treatments available through a local pharmacist, to speak to nurse, to call 111 or 999, or to go to hospital or book appointment
- Prevent infected patients visiting clinics or surgeries
- Reduce angry or demanding patients who may abuse staff
- Relevant information and leaflets are freely distributed
- Able to offer videos, pictures and other help to educate patients
- No additional investment required for infrastructure or special software
- Service very soon available via the Internet and Internet cafés

BENEFIT TO PATIENTS

- Reduces costs of consultation, wasted tests and investigations
- Reduced antibiotic abuse and unwanted drug treatment
- Reduction in travel time and people coming to towns from villages
- Primary health care center in remote area managed by non-medicals
- Reduced cost of telecare and telemedicine
- Reduction in X-Ray report using expensive software or computers
- Encourages patients to reveal common symptoms that may prove to be serious
- Reduce medical errors and complications due to delay
- Helps doctors to investigate and make accurate diagnoses
- Allows patients to easily connect with another doctors and get a second opinion
- Patients from UK, USA and Europe can communicate with doctors in India and people in India can also get second opinion from specialists in other country
- Ease communication with doctors from all over the world
- Reduce cost of prescriptions by allowing patients to get drugs delivered home
- Senior citizens will find video helpful, reduce travel and waiting

Please download our Apps Dr. MAYA and request your doctor to download MAYA Dr from Google Play, Apple Stores and try.

There are more important features we have tested and will be offered if the hospital or department of health requests.

MAYA APP - INSTRUCTION

MAYA WILL NOT DIAGNOSE ANY ILLNESS BUT WILL HELP YOU DIFFERENTIATE MINOR FROM SERIOUS ILLNESS.

Please choose three symptoms to help MAYA decide on the severity of the illness and urgency of treatment required to help you reduce delay and complications.

"If you are very sick and unable to follow the instructions, PLEASE CALL EMERGENCY SERVICE AND GO TO HOSPITAL."

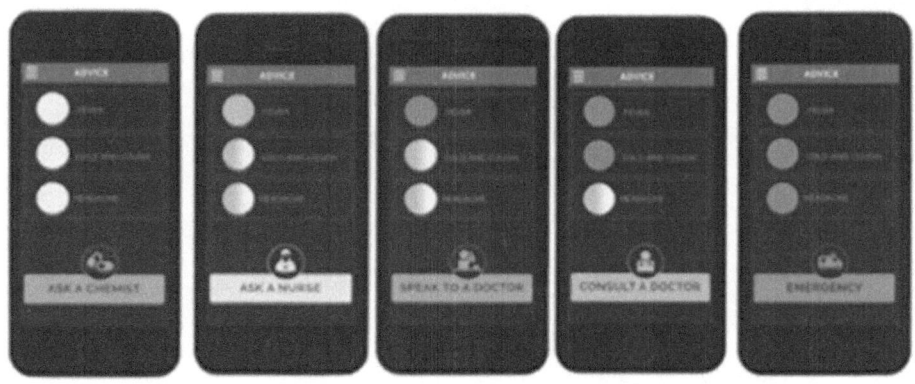

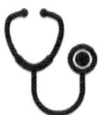 **"THREE RED"**

Please treat the illness as potentially "Serious." A specialist must see you in a hospital, clinically examine, investigate and offer treatment or advice. Visiting doctors or your GP in the surgery will delay in diagnosing and getting the right treatment you need.

Please call emergency number if advised or go to Accident & Emergency (A&E) or Emergency Room (ER) in the local hospital. Doctors visiting you at home will not be able to offer the right treatment because they need to perform investigations. "Please Do Not Drive" to the hospital.

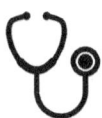 **"TWO RED"**

You must consult a doctor NOW. Doctors in the community may manage the symptoms you choose. Doctors may be clinically trained and have the knowledge and experience to examine you properly, organize tests if necessary and offer the correct treatment.

Please request an emergency appointment in the surgery or go to hospital if you cannot get an appointment to consult a doctor. Doctors will clinically examine, request tests, scans to help them diagnose illness or refer you to specialist.

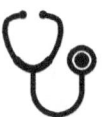 **"ONE RED"**

The symptom you chose is RED, you must speak to a doctor before you book an appointment or go to surgery or hospital. Some doctors may offer advice or prescribe treatment based on the story of your illness. Some doctors will insist on examination but others may opt not to and investigation

Doctors will ask some questions and offer advice or suggest consultation.

 ## "GREEN"

THREE or TWO GREEN Symptoms with YELLOW can be managed by nurses. Please call doctor out of hour's service and speak to a nurse or speak to a doctor.

The symptoms or complaint you choose are common and in UK some surgeries have nurses who are allowed to prescribe medication and advice based on protocol. If your surgery or clinic does not have trained nurses, then please speak to your doctor or go to Accident and Emergency care in hospital.

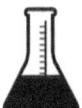 ## "YELLOW"

Illness with Three YELLOW Symptoms can be managed using treatment available in the local chemist. If you are worried and not sure, please call and speak to a doctor.

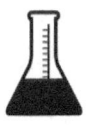 ## NEW SCORING SYSTEM FOR INDIA & OTHER DEVELOPING COUNTRIES

To keep cost of this book down we have resorted to use shades of black and gray. Each symptom has numbers, so please make a note of the number of three symptoms and act based on the total score.

Score: Action

More than 30: Emergency – Go To Hospital/Call Ambulance
Score 21 – 29: Emergency Consultation With Doctor

Score 10 – 20:   Speak To Doctor
Score 0–10:   Consult Chemist

RED: Each symptom must be scored as 10 (Ten)
GREEN: Each Symptom must be scored as 5 (Five)
YELLOW: Each Symptom mustscored as 3 (three)

- R + R + R = 30   EMERGENCY
- R + R + G = 25   CONSULTATION
- R + R + Y = 23   CONSULTATION
- R + G + G = 20   SPEAK TO A DOCTOR
- R + G + Y = 18   SPEAK TO A DOCTOR
- R + Y + Y = 16   SPEAK TO A DOCTOR
- G + G + G = 15   SPEAK TO A DOCTOR OR NURSE
- Y + Y + Y = 09   ASK A CHEMST

INSTRUCTIONS TO SET UP MAYA DR FOR DOCTORS

1. Please note that you are liable for all advice and treatment you offer to patients registered under your name or the registered patient of any Maya Dr network.
2. Fees will be paid as indicated after deducting 20% towards administration and maintaining the database.

DOCTORS SET-UP

1. Register as a doctor in the Maya Dr app
2. Enter your name and your speciality from the drop-down menu. Enter your mobile numbers (including the country code), Medical Council Registration number, Surgery or clinic, country and choose a password.
3. Log-in using your email and password.
4. Click on the drop-down menu on the left side in the next screen.
5. Choose the set-up tab and enter your mobile telephone number, email ID and your Skype name for video and messaging services, press enter to save.
6. Click on "Patients" and add information about your patient and save by clicking/pressing Enter.
7. Click on Patient List to see if the name and contact details of the patient have been stored.

8. Click on the Symptom Button and Add Symptoms using the language of your choice, choose a colour (which denotes the seriousness of the condition) and then enter the relevant information and your advice, plus any URL Link and/or Video. Please note that patients registered in your database will have access only to the database you create and not the master database on the Maya system server.

9. Click on "Notes" during a consultation, enter information into the notes and forward this via email or another messaging service to the email address of the patient.

10. Once you have sent the email, your patient and you will receive a copy of the notes. Maya Dr does not store this information and does not retain access to this data in the future.

11. Doctors can send prescriptions to patients or pharmacists and also send letters of referral to hospitals or specialists.

12. During consultations doctors can also click on the "NHS" or Google buttons to get online information and other help.

2003©KMS | Patent Protected GB1004457.6

COMMON SYMPTOMS

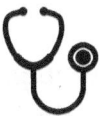 **ABDOMINAL PAIN**

The abdomen is that part of your body which is below your ribs and above your hips. Some people call it the trunk, tummy, belly or gut.

When you have pain in that area, doctors will call it abdominal pain. However, other popular terms for abdominal pain include tummy pain, tummy ache, stomach ache, stomach pain, gut ache, and belly ache.

Pain that you feel here is usually linked to a problem in your gut, but you may be experiencing referred pain from problems existing in your chest or groin.

Pain in the abdomen (tummy pain) is a very common symptom that can be very difficult for doctors to diagnose, and frustrating for affected patients.

This is one of the symptoms that doctors can often get wrong because they have not identified the cause, or have managed the problem without proper clinical examination, or have simply suppressed the symptom using drugs.

Pain in the abdomen usually does not last long and is often due to a gut infection or a small digestive upset – but there are many other possible causes.

Pain that is severe, or doesn't settle quickly, must be examined and managed only by a doctor in the hospital. If not, the chances of long-term complications are very high.

This is one symptom that can take many doctors by surprise, because they forget to examine the chest, abdomen, and groin areas to rule out referred pain. If you are not happy with the doctors or nurses, and feel that they have not listened, or have offered treatment or advice without carrying out a clinical examination of the chest, groin, and abdomen, please consult another doctor.

Different types of pain you may feel are: sharp or stabbing, crimpy, spasmodic, colicky, or a general dull ache. Colicky pain is sharp, spasmodic (on and off), and gradually becoming worse.

Commonly associated symptoms are: fever, constipation, watery diarrhoea, blood or mucus in stool, vomiting, nausea, anorexia, dysuria, and increased frequency of urine.

Tonsillitis, rhinitis, sinusitis, pharyngitis, or otitis media (often labeled as URTI or Upper respiratory tract infection) may cause abdominal pain due to enlarged lymph nodes. This is called mesenteric adenitis but majority of doctors are not convinced. This often gets better on its own.

You may experience coughing, fever, and pain in the chest when you breathe in. These symptoms would suggest that you have a chest infection and must not be anaesthetized. Please make sure the doctor has examined your chest to rule out a chest infection that has produced radiating pain localized in your abdomen. The presence of any pain in your testicles or groin is also important.

Please do not take any medication yourself (pain killers, ibuprofen, etc.), but if you have done, make sure you inform the doctor.

Common causes of abdominal pain are gastritis, gastro-enteritis, trapped wind, diarrhoea, food poisoning, appendicitis, period pain, Irritable Bowel Syndrome, kidney stones, Pelvic Inflammatory Disease, gall stones, and ulcers.

DO NOT PANIC, because anxiety can make this symptom worse.

Please make sure you do not drink or eat if the associated symptoms suggest you go to hospital as an emergency. Please consult doctors or go to a hospital before you take painkillers or other drugs if the other associated symptoms are RED.

Pain that comes on suddenly may be called acute. Longer-standing pain is called chronic.

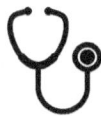 ALTERED STATE OF MIND

If the person looks as if he/she is awake, but they cannot answer simple questions like their name, age, birth date, or where they live, then consider this an "Altered state of mind."

The common causes are drug or alcohol abuse, low blood sugar, dehydration, head injury (early or late complication), and environmental effects.

Extremes in temperature – excess cold or heat – can make people faint or have an altered state of mind.

A rapid increase in body temperature can result in fits (febrile convulsions), or delirium (talking oddly/ in gibberish).

Management:

Give the affected person a high calorie drink such as non-fizzy cola, with one or two pinches of salt for every can or glass, or get them to eat chocolate. This will increase their blood sugar and also fluid levels in the body, and patient will start talking normally.

If the temperature is hot – try tepid sponging (using lukewarm water, not cold or ice cold water). If cold, warm the patient up using blankets, or give them a hug so that you can share your body heat to warm the cold patient (please make sure the person does not have vomit, blood, faeces, saliva or urine on their clothes).

When they wake up and start talking, re-assess.

Ask simple questions, and call their relatives or family members using the telephone.

If the patient is not responding or is losing consciousness, or does not improve within a few minutes, call an ambulance and send the patient to hospital.

AMENORRHOEA

The medical term used to describe "absence of periods."

Women normally do not menstruate before puberty, during pregnancy and after menopause.

If you have stopped or missed having periods, and are sexually active, please consult a chemist and get pregnancy test. Doctors will investigate and offer advice and treatment if you are not pregnant.

There are two types of amenorrhea: primary and secondary amenorrhea. Primary amenorrhea is when a young woman has not had her first period by the age of sixteen. Secondary amenorrhea is when a woman who has had normal menstrual cycles stops getting her monthly period for three or more months.

This is a common and early symptom of stress, depression, and anorexia, and is said to be associated with viral infections. Post-Ebola infected patients are said to experience this as a late complication. Women who were on oral contraceptives may also develop amenorrhoea for a long time.

Please consult a family planning clinic, or speak to a doctor.

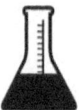
ANKLE PAIN

It is often difficult to differentiate a sprain from a fracture or complete tear of the lateral ligament based on clinical examination.

An X-Ray may help to diagnose severe injuries, with tenderness other than in the ligament area, and where there is instability or undue movement at the joint.

If no fracture or complete tear is suspected, doctors will treat this symptom as a sprained ankle. In the acute phase, treatments include ice, ultrasound (if available) and elevation.

The most common treatments that pharmacists will advise are non-steroid anti-inflammatory analgesics (NSAID) like nitrogen, brufen, voltarol, diclofenac, naproxen with or without Paracetamol, or acetaminophen.

If the pain does not resolve with anti-inflammatory drugs, a doctor will do more tests, investigations and refer you to orthopedics or a rheumatologist. If you are suffering from asthma, tummy pain, gastritis or indigestion, please consult a doctor, and do not take these drugs.

Anti-inflammatory analgesics must not be stopped as soon as you feel the pain has gone. Please continue taking them for two to three days. If you don't, the pain will come back.

Physiotherapy and/or exercise when you have ankle pain is not a good idea, because the inflamed joint is very brittle and may take greater harm. You should exercise or get physiotherapy only after you have taken treatment and the pain has eased.

Strapping and Elastoplast can be used to give support to the ankle, foot, and calf. Please consult a bone specialist (orthopedician) about this treatment.

Severe sprains should be treated in plaster of Paris.

Please note, torn ligaments, if not treated early and managed by a specialist can result in long-term problems.

X-Rays and Ultrasound scans are not useful to diagnose a tear, so you may need an MRI Scan. Please consult a doctor if this symptom is bad and NSAID did not help.

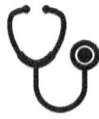
ANKLE SWELLING

Swollen ankles, feet and legs are a common and important symptom that suggests heart failure, abnormal salt, protein, and water balance in the body. Doctors call this oedema.

Swelling associated with pain is likely to be due to traumatic injury, and not necessarily associated with the heart, or retention of fluid in the body.

It is often difficult to separate a sprain, fracture or complete tear of the lateral ligament from oedema based on clinical examination. An X-Ray may be required to help differentiate injuries with tenderness other than in the ligament area and where there is instability or undue movement at the joint. If no fracture or complete tear is suspected, doctors will refer the case, or do tests to rule out serious heart or kidney conditions.

If the swelling is gradual (chronic), pain free and not associated with trauma, elevation of leg will help reduce swelling.

The most common treatment doctors will prescribe is furosemide (water tablets). Please note you will pass large amounts of urine within 2–4 hours and so these are best taken when you are at home, and not just before bedtime.

A doctor will do tests and investigations, and refer to a cardiologist or nephrologist for a second opinion and advice regarding management.

The majority of patients with this symptom or sign will also have ascites (swollen tummy), swollen legs, and maybe hands as well.

You must consult a doctor.

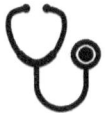 # APHASIA

Aphasia means an inability to speak because of some neurological or psychological problem.

A common cause is laryngitis caused by infections, and if this is the case, you will have associated symptoms to help diagnose this condition.

Friends, family and associates often get worried and rush you to hospital or call in the emergency services.

It can be difficult for doctors, nurses or relatives to identify the cause of aphasia and offer advice. You must consult a doctor to get the correct investigations and diagnosis before treatment.

A stroke, intracranial bleeding, or tumors pressing on the nerves supplying the face, can result in dysarthria (lack of coordination of muscles). Not many people can understand what the patient is talking about. Some people revert back and start speaking in a different language or accent.

This is not a common symptom, but is often associated with vertigo, head injury, alcohol intoxication, neurological problems, drug use, and infections.

As there are numerous causes and they are very difficult to diagnose, specialist help is required.

This may be a presenting symptom of a psychological problem, depression, or simply associated with stress.

Please consult doctors now, or go to hospital.

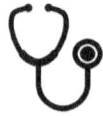 ## ARM NOT MOVING

Toddlers are notorious for often falling and hurting themselves. The first thing you need to rule out is a fracture.

If the child is hyperactive, autistic, or inquisitive, he or she will run around the house or garden, and so it is difficult to be vigilant.

After a fall, the majority of these kids do not cry, because they have an adrenal surge that prevents them from experiencing pain. A few hours after the fall, they may stop moving their arms, or cry as pain starts kicking in.

Some parents may notice swelling, or identify localized pain in the shoulder, arm, elbow or wrist.

This can also happen a few days after the child develops a sore throat caused by a streptococcus infection. This was a common problem, known as "Rheumatic Fever" in the past, but declined after Penicillin became available. The antibodies produced to fight infection suddenly start attacking the joints and heart. Please consult a doctor and make sure to remind him or her about rheumatic fever. We anticipate that this infection may return soon.

Joint pain in children is not rare, and diagnosis depends on the root cause.

It is either poly-articular (multiple joints), mono-articular (one joint), fleeting arthritis, migrating arthritis (spreading from one joint to another or jumping from one joint to another).

Please consult a paediatrician to decide which specialist can help manage this problem. This may be a Rheumatologist or an Orthopedician.

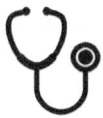 ## ARTHRALGIA

This word is used when you are suffering from various joint pains.

This is a very common symptom that must first be self-treated before consulting a doctor. If you do not, you are wasting time and money.

The most common treatments pharmacists will advise are non-steroid anti-inflammatory analgesics (NSAID) like nurofen, brufen, voltarol, diclofenac, naproxen with or without Paracetamol, or acetaminophen.

The main side effect of these drugs is gastritis and tummy pain. People who have or develop gastritis must consult a doctor and discontinue the treatment.

A family doctor will do tests and investigations, and refer you to orthopedics or a rheumatologist if the pain does not resolve with anti-inflammatory drugs.

Please do not stop the treatment as soon as you feel the pain has gone. Please continue it for two to three days. If you do not, the pain will often return.

Physiotherapy and/or exercise when you have pain is not good, because the inflamed joint is very brittle and might take greater harm. You should exercise or undergo physiotherapy only after you have taken treatment and the pain has eased.

If the problem is chronic, please consult a doctor.

If you experience numbness in your arm, legs, or skin, please treat this as an emergency and consult your doctor today. People often assume numbness is common, and either put off getting the diagnosis and treatment, or self-treat. This is not a good idea, because serious long-term neurological illnesses are often associated with numbness, so please consult a doctor if you have this in association with joint pain.

This symptom is now said to be associated with the Ebola virus.

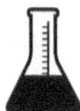 ## ARTHRITIS

This is a very common symptom that must first be self-treated before consulting a doctor. If you do not, you are wasting time and money, because the doctors will first prescribe anti-inflammatory analgesics with or without Paracetamol or acetaminophen.

The main side effect of this NSAID is gastritis, bleeding and tummy pain. People who have or develop gastritis must consult a doctor and discontinue the treatment.

A family doctor will do tests and investigations, and refer you to orthopedics or a rheumatologist if the pain does not resolve with anti-inflammatory drugs.

Please Do NOT stop the treatment as soon as you feel the pain has gone. Continue it for two to three days – if you do not, the pain will often return.

Physiotherapy and/or exercise when you have pain is not good, because the inflamed joint is very brittle and may take greater harm. You should exercise or undergo physiotherapy only after you have taken treatment and the pain has eased. If the problem is chronic, please consult a doctor.

If you experience numbness in your arm, legs, or skin, please treat this as an emergency and consult your doctors today. People often assume numbness is common, and either put off getting the diagnosis and treatment, or self-treat.

This is not a good idea, because serious long-term neurological illnesses are often associated with numbness, so please consult a doctor if you have this in association with joint pain.

This symptom is now said to be associated with the Ebola virus.

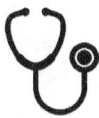 ## ASCITES

When fluid slowly accumulates between the lining of the abdomen wall and the organs, this is known as ascites.

Please note that the distension occurs in periods of short duration. Arms, waist and legs may not be soft, but are often thin.

This is not very common, but is often missed because people assume they are getting obese.

Ascites usually occurs when the liver stops working properly, or the blood pressure in the liver and pancreas increases (portal hypertension). Fluid fills the space between the lining of the abdomen and the organs.

Liver scarring is a common cause of ascites. Scars will increase pressure inside the liver's blood vessels, forcing fluid into the abdominal cavity, and causing ascites.

Liver damage from sources such as cirrhosis, hepatitis B or C infection, alcohol abuse, and heart or kidney failure are the common causes of ascites.

Other conditions that may increase your risk of ascites include: ovarian, pancreatic, liver, or endometrial cancer, pancreatitis, and tuberculosis.

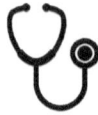 ## ASTHMA

This common illness can potentially become serious.

It is not a disease, but a common illness that can be diagnosed based on a history of illness. The treatments available will not cure you, but will help reduce symptoms like coughing, wheezing, and breathlessness.

Recurrent colds, and coughing that occurs after exercise, running, exposure to cold wind, in the morning, night, and seasonally, must be treated as asthma and investigated.

Most patients assume there are special tests to diagnose asthma.

A peak flow meter can be used to monitor breathing, but this is not a tool that I found useful to diagnose or manage acute asthma. Some patients request a spirometer, but this is expensive and often not required.

Asthma is poorly managed because some doctors, nurses, and patients have not understood the pathophysiology well, and so are prescribing cough mixtures and often misdiagnosing this as a chest infection or LRTI and prescribing antibiotics.

Conflicting opinions and years of abusing antibiotics have made it difficult for doctors like me to manage. Asthma related viral infections often get better on their own, so patients who assume they have an infection also assume the antibiotic worked.

Please note that coughing or feeling breathless at regular intervals is not normal. People believe they catch cold often and the infection goes to their chest, and they demand antibiotics. If you use your common sense, I am sure you will realize that fluid released in the nostrils will drain out through your nostrils when you stand (runny nose, snuffles), but when you lie down, the same fluid will drain down and try to enter your lungs (post nasal drip). The cough is a reflex to protect the lungs, so you will wake up coughing.

If you are someone who has an on and off cough, please consult a doctor who knows what he or she is talking about and will listen to your story and offer the right treatment.

Preventative treatment using mild steroids helps reduce antibiotic abuse.

Please note that drugs used to treat asthma open the airways and prevent them from getting blocked, so you will cough more to clear the sputum (phlegm) from your chest. Only after all the secretions in your lungs are cleared will you stop coughing.

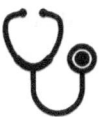 ASTHMATIC COUGH

This cough is usually dry, spasmodic and very distressing, and occurs in patients suffering from asthma, hay fever, and other allergic conditions that produce a dry cough.

This cough is typically wheezy, with a whistling or musical sound.

People with post nasal drip, or who are smokers, often have this cough. The mucus from the sinuses drains down the back of the throat, and the body tries to cough the secretion out. The cough will normally be worse when you lie down, or when you first wake up in the morning.

This is quite common with those who suffer from hay fever although, if an allergy is present that is due to something other than seasonal hay fever, a cough can be present all year round.

Even if you think this is the cause of your morning cough, it is important to have a proper diagnosis made by your doctor.

It is not wise to self-medicate, as many antihistamine preparations will have side effects, and certain types of cough – like an asthmatic or allergic cough – must not be suppressed.

Asthma inhalers open your airways, and the body will have to get rid of the sputum or phlegm that has collected in the lungs. If the dry cough becomes productive – bringing out lots of phlegm, please do not take cough mixtures or think you have an infection. Your technique of inhaling the drug is good, and coughing soon after taking the drug indicates that you are responding to treatment.

If you do not cough more and bring out phlegm or sputum, then please consult your doctor. Your technique may be poor, or you may have an infection that is not allowing the drug to enter your lungs well.

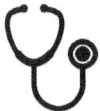 ## ATAXIA

This means irregular, purposeless movement. This is not a common symptom, but may be associated with vertigo, head injury, alcohol intoxication, drugs and infections.

Poor muscle coordination can affect speech, eye movements, hearing, swallowing, walking, picking up objects, and other voluntary movements.

Persistent ataxia may be caused due to damage to the cerebellum, the part of the brain that controls muscle coordination.

Common causes are: The aftermath of brain surgery, head injuries, alcohol abuse, drug abuse, infections such as chickenpox, brain tumors, and the effects of toxic chemicals.

Rarer causes are multiple sclerosis (MS), cerebral palsy, some other neurological conditions, congenital abnormality, or tumors.

Ataxias are named based on location, organ, or the person who first identified the illness. They are: Friedreich's ataxia, spino-cerebellar ataxia, or ataxia-telangiectasia. There are forty (40) types of inherited ataxia listed in medical literature.

Ataxia can affect organs like the eyes (optic ataxia) and lungs (ataxic respiration-uncoordinated respiratory movements, usually due to dysfunction of the respiratory centers of the medulla oblongata).

Cerebellar ataxia can present as floppiness (hypotonic), a lack of coordination between organs, muscles, limbs or joints, an impaired ability to control the distance, power, and speed of an arm, hand, leg or eye movement (dysmetria), an inability to perform rapid, alternating movements (dysdiadochokinesia), and difficulty in accurately estimating time (dyschronometria).

Vestibulo-cerebellum ataxia affects balance, eye movement and control. The patient will typically stand with feet wide apart, in order to gain better balance and avoid swaying backwards and forwards (posterior-anterior oscillations). Even when the patient's eyes are open, balance is difficult when the feet are together.

Spino-cerebellum ataxia presents as an unusual gait, with unequal steps, sideways steps, and uncertain starts and stops.

Cerebro-cerebellum ataxia causes the patient to have problems carrying out voluntary, planned movements. The head, eyes, limbs, and torso may tremble as voluntary movements are carried out. Speech may be slurred, with variations in rhythm and loudness.

Sensory ataxia occurs due to loss of proprioception. Proprioception is the sense of the relative positions of neighboring parts of the body. It is a sense that indicates whether the body is moving with the required effort, and also where the various parts of the body are located in relation to one another.

A patient with sensory ataxia typically has an unsteady, stomping gait, with the heel striking hard as it touches the ground with each step. Instability becomes worse in poorly lit environments. If a doctor asks the patient to stand with eyes closed and feet together his/her instability will clearly worsen. This is because loss of proprioception makes the patient much more reliant on visual data.

The patient may find it hard to perform smoothly coordinated voluntary movements with the limbs, trunk, pharynx, larynx, and eyes.

Some people may develop ataxia without doctors or specialists being able to find out what the cause was.

Symptoms may vary depending on the severity and type of ataxia, of which there are many. If the ataxia is caused by an injury or another health condition, symptoms may emerge at any age, and may well improve and eventually disappear.

Common Symptoms:
- Poor limb coordination resulting in walking difficulties – in severe cases the patient may need a wheelchair.
- Dysarthria – slurred and slow speech. It is difficult to produce sounds, or control the volume, rhythm, and pitch of speech.
- Swallowing difficulties, resulting in choking or coughing.
- Facial expressions become less apparent.
- Limbs and other parts of the body may shake or tremble unintentionally.
- Nystagmus – involuntary rapid, rhythmic, repetitious eye movement. Poor vision results from this, and eye movements may be vertical, horizontal, or circular.
- Pes cavus – a foot with too high an arch.
- Cold feet – because of a lack of muscle activity.
- Problems with balance.

Depression can occur as a result of having to live and cope with these symptoms.

You must consult a doctor (neurologist), because this may be a complication of infection, drugs, or a neurological condition.

This is not a common symptom most GPs encounter, so any delay in diagnosis is not in your interest.

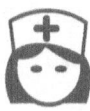
BABY CRYING WHEN FEEDING

Common causes are thrush in the mouth, or difficulty breathing (nose blocked or has breathing difficulties). A baby may find it frustrating to suck a bottle if the teat hole is small. Some babies are constipated, and may often pull their legs up. Always look at the anus of babies to see if there are any fissures or cuts that may bleed. Babies with blocked noses find it hard to suck a bottle or breast. Babies fed on bottle will struggle to breastfeed because sucking from a breast is more straining. If the baby is drifting to sleep when breast-feeding, please make sure the baby has sucked well. Babies struggling to feed often suck in air that fills the stomach. They then wake up and start crying because they are still hungry. Please consult a nurse or midwife for advice.

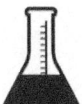
BACK PAIN

This is a very common symptom that must first be self-treated before consulting a doctor. The reason you must try to self-treat is because doctors will first offer the same treatment that a chemist would advise. The first stage in diagnosing the problem (if it is not associated with danger signs) is to rule out common problems.

The most common treatment is anti-inflammatory analgesics like nurofen, brufen, voltarol, and diclofenac, with or without paracetamol. The main possible problem with these is gastritis – tummy pain. People who have or develop gastritis must consult a doctor.

A doctor may request blood tests, X-Rays, scans and investigations, or may refer you to orthopedics or a rheumatologist. A family doctor (GP) must first try to identify the cause in order to make the appropriate referral (orthopedics or Rheumatologist). If the initial differentiation and referral is not correct, the patient will suffer due to a delay in diagnosis and getting the right treatment, and serious complications will occur.

The majority of patients who complain of chronic back pain have pain which continues because they have stopped taking anti-inflammatory drugs as soon as the pain got better. Please do not stop the treatment. Continue for two to three days, or maybe a week. Inflamed joints are slow to resolve.

Undertaking physiotherapy, and/or starting exercise when the pain is severe because of inflammation, is not a good idea. Inflamed joints are very brittle and can be further harmed, resulting in long-term problems. You should start exercise or get physiotherapy only after you have taken treatment to suppress the inflammation and the pain has eased.

Please consult a doctor if you have chronic back pain that is radiating to your legs or groin, urinary symptoms and severe weakness of the legs peripherally, numbness around your anus, or severe constipation. Retention of urine requires an immediate referral to a specialist.

Referred pain from a kidney or gynaecological infection, and from anxiety and depression, can present as backache.

If you are less than 20 years old or more than 60 years old, or have urinary symptoms, severe weakness of the legs peripherally, numbness around your anus, severe constipation, or retention of urine, please treat this as an emergency and consult a doctor.

If you have numbness in or around your anus – back passage – have dribbling urine or are incontinent, please treat this as an emergency and consult your doctors.

People often assume they have sciatica and self-treat chronic back pain.

80% of patients with backache recover in four weeks, with or without treatment. If the pain is not resolved, you must consult a specialist. Simple 'ligamentous' backache will resolve itself if you are not straining the back when lifting. Take anti-inflammatory analgesia and perhaps take a few days off work. Diazepam is a good muscle relaxant, and should be used to supplement the analgesia.

If the pain is mechanical, it may be due to a prolapsed intervertebral disc. This means that the vertebral disc is exerting pressure on the nerve root.

The sonographers who perform scans have labeled prolapsed disc as "Back bone is crumbling." People with backache believe the backbone is actually breaking into bits, and so are very anxious and difficult to manage. Please note, if the vertebra is crumbling you will not be able to walk, and will experience incontinence and loose sensations below the area.

In the case of older patients, there is the possibility of osteoarthritis, osteoporosis, Paget's disease and/or malignant deposits in the spine.

Mechanical backache is likely to be episodic, related to posture, worse on movement, and relieved by rest. Back pain without these features in the young (less than 20 years old) must be investigated. Low back pain and morning stiffness may go on to develop ankylosing spondylitis (bamboo spine or stiff back).

A plain X-Ray is of limited value in the case of mechanical backache pain or disc prolapse, although a 'normal' X-Ray does have a reassuring (placebo effect) effect on the occasional patient.

For the non-mechanical group a plain X-Ray, full-blood count and ESR is advisable, including a prostate-specific antigen for elderly males and an alkaline phosphatase for older patients of either sex.

It is important to do a rectal examination, listen to the chest and feel the breasts of any elderly patient with undiagnosed back pain.

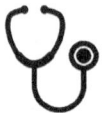 **BARKING COUGH**

Coughing is a symptom we all experience from time to time, and most of us will get over it quickly.

There are many different types of cough, and a barking cough is common in children and some adults. Like many symptoms, a barking cough is often not serious in a child, but a cough that sounds sharp – like a bark – can be very distressing.

The commonest cause is a viral infection, croup (acute trachea-bronchitis) which means the trachea and bronchus are inflamed.

At home, being kept well hydrated will help the child. Also, although there is no real evidence that it works, inhaling moist air does seem to help some children, and you can try that to make them more comfortable. However, if at any point the child appears to be having trouble breathing, you should get him to a doctor as soon as you can.

This symptom often occurs in the early hours of the morning (3–4 am), and is often frightening for parents. This is said to occur because there is a dip in atmospheric pressure at this time, and all respiratory problems get worse.

Doctors do not have any special treatment for this, but will act to prevent dehydration, give analgesics, and observe the patient until they get better. Some children may be treated with inhaled steroids (large doses) to suppress inflammation in the larynx (throat area).

In an adult, a barking cough is an indication that there is swelling in the upper part of the respiratory tract, similar to pharyngitis. This can also occur in children, where if the cough is not too severe it may not be croup.

With children or adults, if you have any doubt you should see the doctor.

As with any complaint that happens suddenly and is not accompanied by a cold, a barking cough should be monitored carefully.

If the cough is accompanied by coughing up blood, or leads to shortness of breath, the child is not feeding or taking fluids, or has any difficulty in breathing then treat this as an emergency and go to A&E.

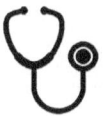

BED WETTING

Known as Enuresis; failure to voluntarily control the passage of urine.

This may occur during the day or night, and 10% of children under 5 years old wet their beds.

Enuresis may be just one of a range of behavioral problems.

Remember to get a urine culture and microscopy test done, to be followed up by a doctor if the test result is abnormal.

Primary enuresis is often due to age or emotional concerns, and Secondary is due to organic causes – a kidney or urinary tract problem, diabetes, or other metabolic problems.

If there are other symptoms, e.g., fever, pain when passing urine (dysuria), increased frequency of urination, or abdominal pain, then think of a urinary tract infection. You must consult a doctor and may need antibiotics. Please note that common bacteria (E. Coli) are now resistant to various antibiotics.

Is the child developing normally, both mentally and physically?

Stresses in the family, changing schools, moving house, or problems in school or nursery will trigger enuresis.

Please do not expect cure for children below the age of 4 years

Consult a health visitor or nurse if a child above 4 years old is wetting the bed, and a doctor if their advice or treatment did not help.

Please make sure that the child does not have a urinary tract infection. If one is present, the treatment must be given as soon as possible to prevent long-term problems.

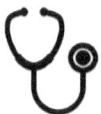 **BEHAVIORAL CHANGE**

This may be how some parents, partners, or carers of children and the elderly explain delirium, talking funny, or being confused.

Diabetic patients may exhibit changes in behavior when their blood sugar is low. It's always safe to try drinking something with sugar or eat some chocolate.

This is a common symptom in the elderly and children with acute viral infections associated with high or very high temperature, and bacterial urinary or chest infections associated with mild to moderate fever, or with feeling hot and cold.

It is also seen in elderly patients who have dementia, Alzheimer's disease, or an occult infection.

Doctors must clinically examine and investigate the patient to rule out other causes of behavior changes.

Common causes are urinary infections, diabetes, dehydration, metabolic disorders, alcohol, the effect of prescription drugs, and drug abuse.

Please do not panic, but go to A&E or the ER if you cannot get an appointment or if you cannot speak to or consult a doctor.

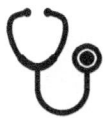

BILE STAINED VOMITING

Bile is green, so green colored vomit is often labeled as bile.

This is a rare symptom, because bile must pass through two valves in order to appear in vomit.

The common causes are intestinal obstruction (intussusception), poisoning, drugs, alcohol, infections, or problems in the liver and gallbladder.

The diagnosis of this symptom requires proper clinical examination, and may require investigation.

Please treat this as an emergency and go to hospital.

Do not panic.

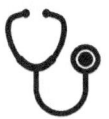

BLEEDING AFTER SEX

This is not a very common problem but occurs in some women. If you are a virgin who had sex for the first time, a vaginal tear, or traumatic injury can produce a slight bleed.

The common causes are menstruation (periods), trauma, infection, thrush, and occasionally a foreign body.

You will need to be examined (vaginally) by doctors to see if you have endometriosis, a foreign body or infections.

The problem is not one that can be managed in your community by a family doctor. Please speak to your doctor and request referral to a gynaecologist.

If the bleeding is severe, please go to hospital now.

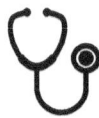 **BLEEDING GUMS**

Sudden onset of bleeding from the mucous membrane in the mouth or gums is common due to blood disorders, nutritional or dietary deficiencies, or damage to the mucus membrane.

This is a major problem seen in patients with the Ebola virus, but bleeding occurred in only half of the patients and is often a late sign.

Please speak to a doctor if you are worried.

If the bleeding is severe, please go to the hospital as an emergency.

Chronic bleeding must be investigated and treated.

Long-term bleeding will produce anaemia and so must be prevented.

Please consult a doctor or a dentist.

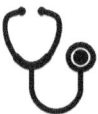 **BLEEDING SPONTANEOUSLY**

Sudden onset of bleeding from mucous membranes (the nose, mouth, vagina or anus), or from intra-venous injection puncture sites is common due to blood disorders, damage to the mucous membrane, and infections.

This is a major problem seen in patients with the Ebola virus.

It is worth noting that in the 1976 Ebola outbreak, bleeding was seen in most cases, whereas in the 1995 Ebola outbreak, bleeding occurred in only half of the patients.

Severe bleeding is a medical emergency, and you must go to hospital.

Bleeding in the arms or legs can be slowed or stopped by applying a tourniquet or bandage that occludes the blood supply.

Please call 999 and go to hospital.

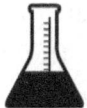

BLOCKED NOSE

This is a very common symptom that is often managed poorly because people do not consult doctors, chemists, or try nasal spray.

Chronic nasal congestion can result in a poor supply of oxygen to brain, resulting in developmental delay and mental retardation in children.

The chronic form is not associated with fever.

The most common cause is allergies. The nasal tissue irritated by allergens (dust, pollens or chemicals) will produce inflammation, resulting in swelling.

Some patients sneeze a lot, and may have a runny nose.

The most common cause of this problem is Hay Fever. This symptom can also occur in winter due to viral infections or colds precipitating inflammation in the nostrils.

Viral infections in the throat, nose, and ears can also produce the same symptom. A watery secretion dripping from the nose is a normal response to trap and wash away dust, allergic triggers or micro-organisms, preventing them from entering the lungs.

We must first help to reduce these secretions by blocking allergens from touching nasal mucosa. Please try self-treatment before consulting a doctor. Doctors who understand pathophysiology will first offer nasal spray, but others may prescribe antibiotics.

The most common treatment is anti-allergy nasal spray.

Try Otrivine Adult Metered Dose 0.1%. Nasal Spray delivers an exact dose of medicated spray inside the nose, and will block production of the secretion. It provides up to 10 hours of relief in as little as 2 minutes. It contains the active ingredient xylometazoline hydrochloride, which helps to open up and clear nasal passages by reducing nasal mucus and returning swollen blood vessels to their normal size. Please note this drug will make the symptom worse if used regularly for more than 3–5 days.

If the problem is chronic, please do not assume you have the common cold. Read all about rhinitis and get the correct treatment. There are a few nasal drops and sprays that can help.

Please note there is no drug that cures rhinitis, but only symptomatic treatments are available – you will stop having this symptom only when you use the nasal spray.

While using a mild steroid spray, you will not have a runny nose or a blocked nose.

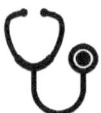 ## BLOOD IN STOOLS

Please note that dysentery is the name used to describe diarrhoea with blood and often mucus in it.

Fresh bloodstain on the toilet roll used to clean your anus is not caused by dysentery, because the stool will be black or tarry (black) colored if the bleeding is in the intestine.

Blood that you may have occasionally noticed dripping into the pan is often due to fissures and/or tears in the anal area.

Constipation, anal sex or trauma can produce tears in the anal region.

This common problem can cause people to panic and rush to hospital.

If the watery stool contains blood and mucus, it is called "dysentery." This is often caused by a worm infestation, amoebiasis, or problems in the intestine.

If the diarrhoea is associated with fever, this may be typhoid. Check the patient's temperature – if it is high and the heart rate is low – and not high as seen in various infections, please ask the doctor to rule out Typhoid.

You may have developed a rose colored rash, and if the blood test is positive, you will need special drugs and hospital care.

You must contact a tropical disease specialist for advice and treatment.

Amoebic dysentery and other intestinal infestations must be investigated.

Please consult a doctor, and get investigations if a tear or fissure is noticed in the anus.

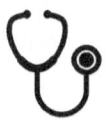 BLOOD IN URINE

Red or dark colored urine frightens people. Passing red colored urine does not necessarily mean that you have a serious problem. First, you need to get your urine checked in the lab.

Beetroot, drugs and some chemicals used in food, as well as infections, can cause urine to go red.

If a nurse or doctors say you have blood in your urine, as determined by the Dipstick test done in surgery, please note that this does not confirm diagnosis. The dipstick has an expiry date, must be stored at room temperature, and is often not accurate.

Doctors will request a microscopic examination to confirm urine has blood in it before they diagnose the cause, and will not assume that it is an infection and start antibiotics.

The most common causes of this symptom are a urinary infection, trauma, bleeding after sex, and kidney stones.

Serious illnesses like post-streptococcus infection, glomerulonephritis, and bladder cancer can also present with blood in urine.

The diagnosis of this symptom requires proper clinical examination, and will require investigations like blood tests and scans.

Please make sure that the doctors check your blood pressure and weight if you have swollen legs or face.

Please do not panic, but go to A&E if you cannot get an appointment or you cannot speak to or consult a doctor.

This symptom must be adequately investigated and treated properly with the right antibiotics.

Doctors and nurses in some countries follow protocols that are now obsolete and therefore unsafe, because a urinary tract infection is now very difficult to clear, as we have run out of antibiotics that kill the bacteria. So you must be careful and avoid contact.

Please do not panic, but go to A&E if you cannot get an appointment, or you cannot speak to or consult a doctor.

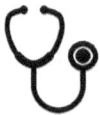 **BLOOD SHOT EYES**

Spontaneous bleed with no associated pain may be associated with high blood pressure or trauma to the eye.

This is known as subconjunctival hemorrhage. The conjunctiva is the thin tissue that covers the sclera. It is the outermost protective coating of the eyeball.

Small blood vessels within the conjunctiva may break spontaneously or from injury, causing a red area on the sclera, and resulting in a subconjunctival hemorrhage.

This appears as a bright red or dark red patch on the white of the eye.

Diagnosis is made on the basis of the appearance of the hemorrhage and the absence of other findings.

Most subconjunctival hemorrhages clear up without treatment in one to two weeks.

Conjunctival blood vessels. Since most subconjunctival hemorrhages are painless, a person may discover a subconjunctival hemorrhage only by looking in the mirror, or by another person seeing a red spot on the white of their eye. In rare cases these may be caused by excessive sneezing, coughing, vomiting and rubbing of the eyes, Contact lenses and conjunctivitis are common causes.

Treatment is symptomatic, using antibiotics if bacterial infection is suspected.

If this symptom does not resolve, you may need blood tests and investigation. Please consult a doctor.

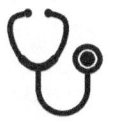 BLUE COLORED FINGERS AND TOES

This is what we call peripheral cyanosis. The most common causes are poor circulation and cold, and this is also seen in some smokers. This symptom is associated with heart, chest and circulation problems. You need to consult a doctor to see if there is any condition that requires treatment.

Bluish discoloration around cut, open wounds, or after suturing, can be due to wound inflammation associated with poor circulation.

Infection can also cause the edges to be blue, but you will have other associated symptoms in this case.

If pus or watery discharge is seen, the wound may have an infection. Please do not delay in consulting a doctor. The bacteria that infect wounds are resistant to treatment.

Taking antibiotics orally or using antibiotic creams, ointments, or alcohol wash can do more harm than good.

Please speak to or consult a doctor.

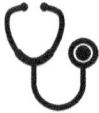 BLURRED VISION

Acuteness, clearness, or sharpness of vision depends on optical and neural factors to focus the eye.

It depends on the retina, and the sensitivity of the interpretative faculty of the brain.

A common cause of low visual acuity is refractive errors, or errors in how the light is refracted in the eyeball.

Causes of refractive errors include aberrations in the shape of the eye ball or cornea, and loss of flexibility in the lenses. These aberrations may be caused by muscle spasms.

Too high or too low refraction (an error in relation to the length of the eyeball) is the cause of near-sightedness (myopia) or far-sightedness (hyperopia). Other optical causes are astigmatism or more complex corneal irregularities.

These anomalies can mostly be corrected by eyeglasses, contact lenses, or laser eye surgery. As part of various medical or neurological conditions you can develop these problems and experience temporary visual loss or blurring.

This symptom is now common in various emerging infections like Ebola. Please speak to a doctor if you have developed this symptom associated with other common symptoms suggestive of infection.

If you have blurred vision with photophobia and a small pupil, you must go to an eye clinic now.

Treatment with steroid and atropine eye drops will help reduce the threat to sight but is not a cure.

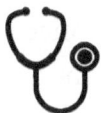

BLUISH COLOR AROUND WOUND

Open wounds and recently sutured wounds can have bluish discoloration around them when the wound is raw or fresh. Infection will also cause the edges to be blue, but you will have other associated symptoms. If pus or watery discharge is visible, the wound may be infected. Please do not delay in consulting a doctor. Bacteria that infect wounds are resistant to treatment. Taking antibiotics orally or using antibiotic creams, ointments or alcohol wash can do more harm than good. Please speak to or consult a doctor.

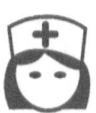

BOTH EYES ARE RED

When both eyes are red, hot, sticky and/or painful, you must consult a nurse or speak to a doctor. This is inflammation of the conjunctiva – the outermost layer of the eye – and of the inner surface of the eyelids.

This most commonly occurs when dust, allergens, irritants or foreign bodies enter the eyes.

Bacterial or viral infections are one of the causes, but need not be the one and only cause that requires any treatment.

Bacterial infections are commonly unilateral (affecting one eye), and will spread to other eye if they are not adequately treated.

Bilateral conjunctivitis is more common in viral infections.

This is said to be an early symptom seen in patients suffering from an Ebola infection.

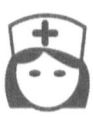 ## BREAST LUMP IN TEENAGER

This is a very common problem in teenagers, and may be noticed in one breast or both. The reason this happens is because hormonal changes during puberty affect boys and girls.

Female hormones are produced and are changed to the male hormone testosterone.

The lumps are painless but boys are often embarrassed.

There is no specific treatment other than investigation of hormone levels.

If there is a lump in one breast, it is better to speak to your doctors and decide what to do.

Some boys have also been reported to secrete milk.

Please speak to a nurse and book an appointment with doctors if she advises you to.

This is not an emergency.

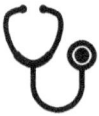 ## BREAST LUMP

If you have felt a lump in your breast, or any other part of the body, you will be anxious.

Painless, soft lumps felt superficially on the breast are common. These are likely to be made of fatty tissue, and are called lipomas.

Hard, irregularly shaped lumps felt under the skin in breast tissue must be seen and examined by a doctor. If you have a history of breast cancer in your family, please consult a doctor soon.

Breast lumps felt on the lower and outer quadrants of both breasts may be due to a bra with metal supports rubbing the soft breast tissue. This can be avoided if you use a sports bra with no metal rings attached.

Breast engorgement and pain can be associated with pregnancy and experienced during periods.

During their teenage years, boys may find that one or two breasts start to enlarge. This is known as Gynaecomastia. Breast development in teenage boys is common during puberty. If pain is present, the ducts may be secreting milk or, if he has a fever (often mild and may cause feelings of heat and cold), there may be an infection.

If one breast is enlarged, you must consult a doctor to rule out other causes of breast enlargement.

Please check if there is milk, turbid fluid, or a blood stained secretion coming out from the nipples.

Have you recently sustained a blunt injury? Bleeding inside the breast (Haematoma) can result in swelling and pain, but not fever. Simple analgesics will help to reduce pain, and ibuprofen can help reduce swelling. Please do not give ibuprofen if the patient is allergic or has gastritis – on and off abdominal (tummy) pain. This drug is taken after food, 3 to 4 times a day.

Obese children and alcoholics often have gynaecomastia.

Please speak to a nurse or a doctor before you book an appointment to consult a doctor, because this is not an emergency.

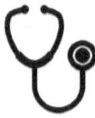 **BREAST PAIN**

If you have felt pain in one breast you will be anxious.

Painful soft lumps with clear margins felt superficially on the breast are common. These are likely to be abscesses.

Hard lumps with clear margins felt under the skin in breast tissue must be seen and examined by a doctor. You may have a collection of loculated breast milk, blood or pus that must be treated with antibiotics or drained. Fever is likely to be an associated symptom (often mild and may cause feelings of heat and cold).

Have you recently sustained a blunt injury? Bleeding inside the breast (Haematoma) can result in swelling and pain, but not fever. Simple analgesics will help to reduce pain, and ibuprofen can help reduce swelling. Please do not take ibuprofen if you are allergic or have gastritis – on and off abdominal (tummy) pain. This drug is taken after food, 3 to 4 times a day.

Breast lumps felt on the lower and outer quadrants of both breasts may be due to a bra with metal support rubbing the soft breast tissue. This can be avoided if you use a sports bra with no metal rings attached.

Breast pain and enlargement can be associated with pregnancy, and experienced during periods.

During their teenage years, boys may find that one or two breasts start to enlarge. This is known as Gynaecomastia. Breast development in teenage boys is common during puberty.

If one breast is enlarged, you must consult a doctor to rule out other causes of breast enlargement.

Please check if there is milk, turbid fluid, or a blood stained secretion coming out from the nipples.

Obese children and alcoholics often have gynaecomastia.

Please speak to a nurse or a doctor before you book an appointment to consult a doctor, because this is not an emergency.

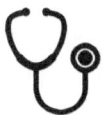 ## BREATHING DIFFICULTY IN ADULTS

This is a common complaint but potentially life threatening, and it is difficult for a doctor to give advice over the telephone, or a diagnosis after clinical examination in primary care.

If the symptom is associated with other symptoms such as severe chest pain lasting more than 15 minutes, vomiting, or pain radiating to the jaw or arms, please call an ambulance and go to hospital.

Sudden onset of breathlessness is not a common symptom.

Chest infections caused by bacteria are often present with mild to moderate fever, followed by breathlessness and no cough. The proper name of this chest infection is pneumonia. It must be treated as an emergency and not with oral antibiotics at home.

Infections in the chest caused by bacteria must be treated with large doses of antibiotics to kill the bacteria. Doctors in the hospital will often start treatment using intra-venous antibiotics given in large doses.

Antibiotics given by mouth are poorly absorbed, and so will only kill the good bacteria and provide an opportunity for resistant bacteria to grow.

Anxiety attacks, panic, and stress can also make some people complain of difficulty in catching their breath and air hunger. They often have associated symptoms like palpitations (audible heart sounds), tachycardia (increased heart rate), and a tingling sensation in their fingers and/or toes.

If this symptom is acute and you feel dizzy, please call 999 and ask for an ambulance to take you to hospital. Please do not drive.

Asthma, chest infections, septicaemia, aspiration, diabetes, and acidosis are some of the common conditions that can cause breathlessness. These are illnesses that can only be managed in hospitals.

This symptom is often associated with other red symptoms, but please treat this as an emergency and consult a doctor even if this happens to be the only red symptom. Please go to A&E or the ER immediately.

If this symptom is associated with other symptoms such as severe chest pain lasting more than 15 minutes, vomiting, or pain radiating to the jaw or arms – please call an ambulance and go to hospital.

Atypical bacteria or viruses can cause breathlessness without any other sign of chest infection. MERS (Middle East Respiratory Syndrome) is a severe, pneumonia-like respiratory disease caused by a virus. It is different from SARS, because MERS is caused by another subtype of the virus. Pneumonia is a general term for an inflammation of the air sacs of the lungs caused by an infection or chemical. With pneumonia, the lungs fill with fluid, which interferes with their ability to transfer oxygen to the blood. MERS is known as an atypical pneumonia because it is not caused by the usual bacteria or viruses. MERS is typically associated with a high fever (over 38°C or 100.4°F), cough, severe shortness of breath, and diarrhoea. The infection is thought to be spread by close contact with an infected person. A virus called coronavirus is the cause of MERS. There are many kinds of coronavirus, some of which cause the common cold. The MERS coronavirus (MERS-CoV) is a new variant that was discovered in 2012 in the Middle Eastern region. How MERS spreads is not completely understood, but experts believe that the main way it spreads is through close contact with an infected person (by caring for or living with the person, or having direct contact with their respiratory secretions and body fluids). The people who have been infected by MERS have all been in a health care facility or among close family members. MERS is different from SARS. Most importantly, the MERS virus does not appear to be as easily spread between people, whereas the SARS virus spreads very easily. Please speak to a doctor before rushing to a clinic, surgery, or hospital. Your doctors will give advice on what you must do.

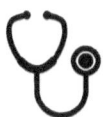 ## BREATHING DIFFICULTY IN CHILDREN

Please do not waste time trying to find out what is wrong with your child and delay consulting a doctor. This is not a common symptom, and you must consult a doctor now.

Please treat this as an emergency symptom even if this happens to be the only symptom that is red. Go to hospital now, and consult a doctor in hospital. This symptom is potentially serious.

Do not go to a walk-in-clinic, primary care, emergency clinic, call 111 to discuss the situation with a nurse, or wait to speak to a doctor. If the symptom is very acute (sudden onset), please call an ambulance. Do not drive to hospital with a child who is breathless.

You must treat this as an emergency and consult a doctor in the hospital, not expect a doctor to visit your home to offer treatment.

Doctors in the hospital will clinically examine the child, and may request a chest X-Ray or scan, perform blood tests, and admit the child for observation in the hospital after diagnosis.

There are numerous causes for this symptom, but none can be safely managed at home. The most common causes are foreign body aspiration, pneumonia and septicaemia, metabolic disorders producing acidosis, diabetes, endocrinal causes, pneumothorax, asthma, an allergic reaction, an anxiety attack, heart failure, and some viral infections.

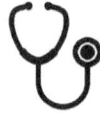 ## BREATHING FAST

Rapid breathing is a condition known as tachypnia. The normal respiratory rate in adults varies between 12 and 20 breaths per minute. Tachypnia is indicated by a ventilator rate greater than 20 breaths per minute. Children have significantly higher resting ventilator rates, which decline rapidly during the first three years of life and steadily thereafter, until they are around 18 years old.

Common causes of tachnypnia are anxiety attacks, metabolic disorders, high fever, infections, metabolic acidosis, diabetes, aspiration, and hormonal problems.

You may feel as if you are about to faint (lose consciousness), hear your heart beating fast (palpitations), and feel a tingling sensation in your fingers and feet, or generalized all over the body. This is typical of a panic attack or anxiety attack.

Try placing a paper or plastic bag over your mouth and nose, and slowly breathing in and out into the bag to see if the symptoms resolve. If you feel better, then this symptom is likely due to an anxiety attack.

This symptom can also be related to a problem in the heart or lungs.

You must consult a doctor as soon as possible, because this symptom is associated with serious illnesses that need to be managed by doctors in the hospital.

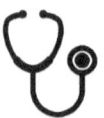 ## BREATHLESSNESS WHEN SLEEPING

Known as orthopnoea, this could be an acute or on-going problem.

People complain of acute breathlessness or feeling as though someone is sitting on their chest and trying to strangulate them.

This is a very frightening symptom, and patients often get very anxious and frightened.

Is a very common symptom of congestive heart failure (heart failure due to a weak heart). Patients will also have associated symptoms that can help a doctor diagnose this illness and offer the right treatment.

They will often have breathlessness when walking, and notice their feet and abdomen are swollen. Such a patient may be on Furosemide (water tablets), and may be a known patient with heart problems.

Please take extra water tablets and speak to a doctor, a cardiologist, or go to hospital if this symptom has occurred for the first time. If you are diagnosed with congestive cardiac failure (CCF), your doctor can help manage your symptoms at home.

If the symptom has occurred for the first time, or is associated with chest pain, blue lips, and feeling anxious, please call 999 and go to hospital as an emergency.

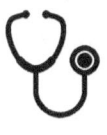 ## BREATHLESSNESS WHEN WALKING UP HILL

This is not a common symptom, and must be seen by a doctor in the hospital, investigated, and treated as an emergency.

In a typical case, this is suggestive of Angina, and may be an early sign of a heart attack. If you are diabetic, you may not have chest pain or other symptoms that will make you rush to hospital. Please go to hospital and consult a doctor now if this symptom has occurred for the first time.

Do not waste time by hoping the symptom will get better on its own, or book an appointment in the surgery to consult a doctor.

The doctors in the hospital must clinically examine you, request routine blood tests, an ECG or EKG (Electrocardio gram), an angiogram, and offer treatment.

Please do not drive. Call an ambulance if the associated symptoms are red, and treat this as an emergency.

Book an appointment in the surgery and consult a doctor if this symptom has been going on for some time and you are already taking treatment for angina. Please make sure you take the GTN Spray as advised by the doctors if the pain is bad.

You may be on aspirin; if you are, you can take another aspirin 300 mg tablet.

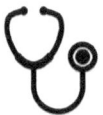 BREATHLESSNESS

This is a common complaint explained by some patients as catching breaths, inability to breathe, air hunger, or a tight chest.

This is a difficult symptom for a doctor to give advice on over the telephone, because you must be clinically examined, and may need a chest X-Ray, scan and other tests to confirm the diagnosis.

If the symptom is associated with other symptoms such as severe chest pain lasting more than 15 minutes, vomiting, and pain radiating to the jaw or arms, please call an ambulance and go to hospital.

Sudden onset of breathlessness is not a common symptom, and must always be treated as a medical emergency.

Chest infections caused by bacteria are often present with mild to moderate fever, followed by breathlessness and no cough. The proper name of chest infection is "pneumonia," and it must be treated as an emergency.

Oral antibiotics are not the right treatment, and you should not start a course of them. You will need intra-venous antibiotics given in large doses. Antibiotics given by mouth are poorly absorbed and so will only kill the good bacteria and provide an opportunity for resistant bacteria to grow.

Anxiety attacks, panic, and stress can also make some people complain of difficulty in catching breath or air hunger, and often creates associated symptoms like palpitations (audible heart sounds), tachycardia (increased heart rate), and a tingling sensation in the fingers and/or toes.

If the symptom is acute and you feel dizzy, please call 999 and ask for an ambulance to take you to hospital. Please do not drive.

Asthma, chest infections, aspiration and acidosis are some of the common conditions that can cause breathlessness. These are illnesses that can only be managed in hospitals

This symptom is often associated with other red symptoms, but please treat this as an emergency and consult a doctor even if this happens to be the only red symptom. Please go to A&E or the ER.

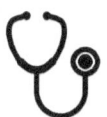 BREATHLESSNESS IN MERS AREA

Middle East Respiratory Syndrome (MERS) is a severe, pneumonia-like respiratory disease caused by a virus. It is different from SARS, because MERS is caused by another subtype of the virus, and similar to mycoplasma producing atypical pneumonias.

Pneumonia is a general term for an inflammation of the air sacs of the lungs caused by an infection or chemical. With pneumonia, the lungs fill with fluid, which interferes with their ability to transfer oxygen to the blood. MERS, mycoplasma, and pneumocystis produce an atypical pneumonia because the air sacs are not filled with sputum, but the walls are thickened, preventing oxygen from passing through.

You will have a high fever, dry cough, and severe shortness of breath. The infection is thought to be spread by contact with an infected person.

A virus called coronavirus is the cause of MERS. There are many kinds of coronavirus, some of which cause the common cold. The MERS coronavirus (MERS-CoV) was a new variant that was discovered in 2012 in the Middle East.

How MERS spreads is not completely understood, but experts believe that the main way it spreads is through close contact with an infected person (by caring for, or living with, the person or having direct contact with their respiratory secretions and body fluids).

The people who have been infected by MERS so far have all been in a health care facility or among close family members.

MERS is different from SARS. Most importantly, the MERS virus does not appear to be as easily spread between people, whereas the SARS virus spreads very easily.

The main symptoms of MERS are: a dry cough, shortness of breath and difficulty breathing, diarrhoea, and high fever (over 38°C or 100.4°F).

PLEASE CONTACT AN ISOLATION HOSPITAL OR CALL THE EMERGENCY MERS HELP LINE. DO NOT GO TO A HOSPITAL OR CLINIC. THE ISOLATION UNIT WILL SEND DOCTORS AND AN AMBULANCE.

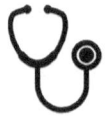 **BRIGHT LIGHT HURTS THE EYE**

The common medical term used for this is Photophobia (fear of light). It is an abnormal intolerance to light, the fear of discomfort or pain to the eyes due to light exposure, or the presence of actual physical sensitivity of the eyes.

Common causes are allergic conjunctivitis and serious illnesses like meningitis. Other causes are migraines, headaches, cataracts, a brain injury, uveitis, blepharitis, coloboma, congenital abnormalities, corneal ulcers, conjunctivitis, injury, allergic conjunctivitis, or infections such as chalazion.

The cause and trigger factor must be identified before treatment is offered.

This can be caused due to conditions related to the eyes or nervous system, for example: too much light entering the eye due to a damaged cornea (corneal abrasion), retinal damage, or pupil(s) unable to normally constrict (seen in cases of damage to the oculomotor nerve). This is also seen in albinism (a lack of pigment in the iris), where the irises can't completely block light from entering the eye.

Patients with photophobia will avoid direct light, and may seek the shelter of a dark room or wear sunglasses.

Please do not panic, but go to A&E or the ER if you think you or a child is unwell, and you cannot get an appointment in surgery or speak to a doctor.

If this symptom has a sudden onset, and the associated symptoms are red, please do not waste time asking for a nurse triage service or expecting doctors to visit you at home. Go to hospital and consult an eye specialist to help get a diagnosis and the right treatment.

 ## BURNING SENSATION WHEN PASSING URINE

The common term used by doctors for this symptom is "Dysuria" because of the pain associated with passing urine.

Women often assume this symptom is cystitis, and try to fight the symptom by drinking water, Cranbury juice or electrolyte powders that help change the pH of urine to make it less irritating to vaginal mucosa.

Unfortunately, antibiotic resistant bacteria that do not respond to treatment now threaten us. Reducing delay in establishing the diagnosis and getting treatment early is essential. Please make an appointment with the nurse and get your urine checked early to help reduce future complications.

Please make sure you get your blood pressure checked regularly.

Babies and children may not complain of pain or burning sensations, but will often scream when opening the bowel, or develop constipation.

New-born babies and infants who start to vomit must be investigated for a urinary tract infection, and investigated to rule out congenital abnormalities in the kidney, urinary bladder, and genitalia.

Adults and children may have associated symptoms such as fever, feeling hot and/or cold, behavioral changes, delirium, chills and rigors, increased frequency or inability to pass urine (anuria). To confirm the diagnosis you will need a urine culture and microscopy.

If blood and proteins are present in urine, the nitrate test is often positive. But if the infection is tested for early, this test may be negative. Please note that this test does not always confirm or rule out the presence of infection, and so must not be relied upon. Patients have developed serious septicaemia because they did not receive the right treatment early.

Please do not waste time before starting treatment if you have all the symptoms that suggest a urinary tract infection, but please make sure you have collected and sent a sample of urine off for testing (microscope and culture sensitivity) in the laboratory.

E.Coli is a common cause of this symptom, and we know the majority of its organisms are resistant to treatment. It has become very difficult to manage these common infections.

If symptoms like fever, and pain when passing urine are not better after taking three doses of antibiotics, please consult your doctor and do not go back to the nurses' clinic or a walk-in-clinic.

You must check the lab results before changing the antibiotics or getting admitted to hospital for intra-venous antibiotic treatment.

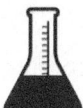 ## BUZZING NOISE IN EARS

A common cause of this is a blockage, or impacted wax in one or both ears.

Infections, and fluid collection behind the eardrum due to sinus congestion, can also produce buzzing and hissing noises.

Try steam inhalation, nasal decongestion, or eardrops to clear the wax first. Ask a chemist for help.

If you are a person who uses ear buds to clear wax, it is likely that you have wax, or otitis external (an infected ear canal) if your ears are itchy.

We see patients demanding consultations for this, and demanding antibiotics or syringing. Neither of these treatments is in your interest, so it is best to avoid abusing antibiotics. Speak to a chemist and get treatment.

Is a constant irritating noise or ringing sound heard in one or both ears? Tinnitus involves the annoying sensation of hearing sounds defined as ringing, buzzing, roaring, clicking, or hissing, that may be present all the time, or may come and go.

Please consult doctors if you develop tinnitus after an upper respiratory infection, such as a cold, and your tinnitus doesn't improve within a week; or if you experience a sudden onset of tinnitus, or if it occurs without an apparent cause.

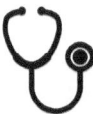 ## CANCER

The word cancer kindles up emotions and makes patients very anxious.

You must know that this is a very rare condition and often has no symptoms.

Patients with cancer often delay their consultation because although they are aware of their condition, they are too scared to consult a doctor and get their diagnosis confirmed.

The majority of lumps and bumps you feel or see on your body are likely to be benign (non-cancerous).

If you are a patient with cancer, on chemotherapy, radiotherapy, or immunosuppressed you must first check associated symptoms.

Do not rush to consult a doctor in the hospital or surgery, because you may get an infection from other patients in the waiting room.

Speak to a doctor first if the other symptom is not RED.

If MAYA suggest you must go to hospital, please call 999, and inform them that you are a patient on drugs for cancer.

Make sure you are not made to wait in A&E but sent to an isolation ward or room to prevent you coming in contact with other patients.

Antibiotic resistant bacteria and emerging viral infections make you vulnerable, and infections are difficult to treat.

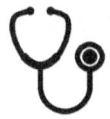

CANNOT BEAR TO SEE BRIGHT LIGHT

The common medical term used for this is Photophobia (fear of light).

The diagnosis of this symptom requires proper clinical examination, and may require investigation.

Common causes are allergic conjunctivitis and serious illnesses like meningitis.

Doctors will only treat this symptom after ruling out serious illnesses, so you must consult a doctor and get a funduscopic examination (an examination of the rear of the eye using an ophthalmoscope).

Please do not panic, but go to A&E or ER if you think you or a child is unwell, and you cannot get an appointment in surgery or speak to a doctor.

Please do not waste time by asking a nurse triage service, calling 111, or expecting doctors to visit you at home.

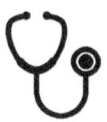

CHEST PAIN

This is not a common symptom, but must be treated as an EMERGENCY.

Severe chest pain lasting more than 15 minutes, not relieved by antacid, associated with vomiting or pain radiating to the jaw or arms must be treated as a myocardial infarction (MI), and managed in hospital.

Please do not waste time trying to find out by yourself what is wrong with you and thus delay in consulting a doctor.

You will need to be clinically examined by doctors, investigated, and either treated or admitted to hospital after diagnosis.

If you do not have any other symptoms that are red, please speak to a doctor and then follow his or her advice.

There are a few common conditions that are associated with chest pain, but the most serious one that it is associated with is a heart attack.

The earlier you get the treatment, the better off you are, because complications often kill patients.

Please take a 300 mg tablet of aspirin if you are not allergic to aspirin. This is said to reduce mortality, and is harmless.

We have seen doctors working in primary care who claim to be experts on interpreting ECG (EKG). They have made simple errors that resulted in deaths. Unfortunately, these errors cannot be identified, and so the problem has been going on for years and these doctors get off scot-free.

We strongly recommend that you go to A&E or the ER of your local hospital and consult a cardiologist to rule out MI (Myocardial Infarction or Heart Attack).

Please call 999 and request an ambulance, or ask someone to drive you to hospital if the hospital is very near. PLEASE DO NOT DRIVE YOURSELF.

Please do not wait to consult your doctors, call an emergency doctor to visit, go to a nurse, or expect visiting doctors to treat you at home.

If you are a patient on treatment for heart problems, or known to have high blood pressure, please treat this as an emergency even if you do not have associated symptoms that are red.

Diabetic patients may not experience chest pain even when they have massive infarctions, so, as we have made clear – Diabetic patients must not use MAYA as a tool to help them learn about their symptoms.

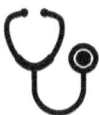 ## CHEST PAIN WHEN BREATHING IN

The diagnosis of this symptom requires proper clinical examination by a specialist in hospital, and may require investigation.

The most common cause of this symptom is pleuritis (inflammation of the membrane covering the lungs), but the problem may also be in the ribs, lungs, or muscles.

Doctors must listen to your chest, and may require a chest X-Ray or scan to rule out pleuritis or effusion (collection of fluid) before starting any treatment.

You may need high dose antibiotics given intravenously.

Blind treatment of this symptom often results in long-term illness. Good doctors will only treat this after ruling out serious illness so you must consult a DOCTOR. Please do not panic. Go to A&E. Please do not waste time waiting to speak to your doctor, or demanding a home visit.

This symptom must be diagnosed and treated in hospital.

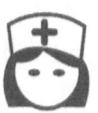 ## CHESTY COUGH

A cough is the our body's response to irritants like inhaled smoke or dust and is there to keep our airways clear of mucus.

Coughing is a reflex and not a disease that can be cured with antibiotics.

Patients complain of coughing out large amounts of phlegm or sputum as a chesty cough, and expect doctors to prescribe them antibiotics. But coughing and the production of phlegm or sputum in a chest infection (Pneumonia), is a sign of you getting better. You cough out sputum (dead bacteria, tissue and white cells in secretion) to clear the air sacs.

A cough is not the main presenting symptom of chest infection – this is breathlessness and/or grunting.

The medical term used by doctors to refer to a chest infection is "Pneumonia." The terms LRTI (lower respiratory tract infection), and URTI (Upper Respiratory Tract Infection) were invented by family doctors within the last two decades to make it easier for people like you to accept antibiotics.

There is actually not a lot of evidence to say that cough medicines do much good, but they will certainly prolong the illness. Honey and lemon, cough mixtures, and aromatherapy were used in the past to help TB patients to liquefy their thick secretions, and so it is not a good idea to use these if you are already coughing up sputum. This cocktail of drugs and mucolytic agents actually paralyzes the diaphragm for some time (suppresses coughing), allowing more time for the secretions to accumulate, so you tend to cough out more sputum when the effect of the drugs wear off.

You must know that coughing is actually a good thing, because the mucus that is produced in the lungs is being coughed out to clear our lungs. In the normal way of things the cough and/or cold that has given rise to the chesty cough will pass, but if it does not then you will have to see the doctor.

You may have to be referred to a respiratory specialist by your doctor if there is no obvious cause for a lingering chesty cough.

You may also need a chest X-Ray to find out what is going on in your lungs. Doctors will often send sputum samples for testing to identify the cause, so that they can give you the right antibiotic if an infection is present.

A chesty cough will normally resolve on its own. If it does not, then you must contact your doctor. Contact your doctor if you also have symptoms that are red, so that doctors can investigate this, offer an accurate diagnosis, and advise treatment.

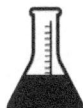 ## CHICKEN POX

If other children in the area had chicken pox, the chances of your child or you getting chicken pox are high. Children exposed to the virus develop chicken pox 7 to 21 days later. Chicken pox typically presents with round small lumps with slight turbid fluid inside. You can find images of these published on the Internet.

In most cases, there are no symptoms before the rash appears. However, a mild fever, stomach ache, and general malaise can occur a day or two before the flat, red rash appears. This generally begins on the scalp, face and back, but can spread to any bodily surface – although it is rarely seen on the palms of the hands or soles of the feet. Lesions are often present in the mouth, and vagina. Intensely itchy, tiny, clear blisters soon follow. Fresh red spots are usually seen next to blisters and crusts.

Most children are free from chicken pox in less than two weeks.

This virus spreads quickly, especially between children. Sneezing, coughing, contaminated clothing, and direct contact with open blisters are all ways of catching this relatively harmless infection.

Complications are very rare, although chicken pox can occasionally lead to encephalitis (inflammation of the brain), meningitis or pneumonia.

Serious complications are more common in children who are on medicines such as steroids, as they can lower the body's immune defense system. Speak to your doctor's surgery for advice now if this is the case.

Treatment is only symptomatic. Use cool baths without soap every three to four hours for the first couple of days. Add a few tablespoons of sodium bicarbonate to the bath water.

Calamine lotion will give temporary relief.

Cotton socks on inquisitive hands will prevent too much scratching, which can lead to infection.

Paracetamol (e.g., Calpol) helps to reduce the fever. Do not give aspirin to children under 12 years of age.

Chicken pox is no longer infectious once 5 days have passed from the time the spots appeared. The child may then return to school.

Please speak to a chemist and get treatment.

Visiting surgery and A&E or the ER is not a good idea because your child or you may catch another infection. You may also infect other patients who are in the waiting area. If you are worried, speak to your doctors or call 111.

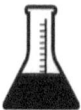 ## CHICKEN POX RASH

Chicken pox typically produces round small lumps with slight turbid fluid inside. You can find images published on the Internet.

This rash may be found in the mouth, vagina and on the tip of the penis, and is very itchy as it starts crusting. If other children in the area had chicken pox, the chances of your child or yourself getting chicken pox is high.

Treatment is only symptomatic. Calamine lotion gives temporary relief. Cotton socks on inquisitive hands will prevent too much scratching, which can lead to infection.

Paracetamol (e.g., Calpol) helps reduce the fever, and antihistamine can reduce the itching. Do not give aspirin to children under 12 years of age.

Please speak to a chemist and get treatment. Visiting surgery and A&E or the ER is not a good idea, because your child or you may catch another infection. You may also infect other patients who are in the waiting area. If you are worried, speak to your doctors or call 111.

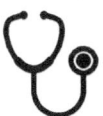 ## CHILLS AND RIGORS

This is a common symptom that is often associated with bacterial infections that can rapidly get worse. You feel hot, cold, and shiver; so this is called Chills and Rigors.

You must consult a doctor and get the correct diagnosis and antibiotics.

It's likely that the infection is in the blood stream, and so may result in septicaemia. Serious common bacterial infections (urinary tract infection, pneumonia, appendicitis, meningitis and glomerulonephritis) all present with history of mild, moderate fever or feeling hot and cold.

Unfortunately, emerging viral infections are also mimicking this symptom.

Please do not panic, but go to A&E if you cannot get an appointment, find a doctor to speak to, or consult a doctor.

This is an early symptom of emerging infections caused by viruses like Ebola.

It is important to let the doctor know your symptoms before visiting any healthcare centers. Infections are spread by contact, and so you may catch another infection or pass on yours to doctors, nurses and other patients at the center.

The majority of patients will require hospitalization, IV antibiotics, and IV fluids. You may require high doses of antibiotics so that the amount entering the blood stream will be high enough to kill the bacteria. If low dose antibiotics are prescribed, the bacteria will hide or develop resistance.

Please consult another doctor if you feel the doctors or nurses are not listening to you. In thirty years, I have seen too many patients become critically ill because the nurses or GPs have reassured them and either treated this as a viral infection or prescribed low dose antibiotics.

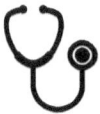

CHOKING

Was the child playing or eating food? The most likely cause is a foreign body, or food particles going into the wrong tube – the air way.

Do not try to look inside the mouth or make the child cry. The foreign particle will only be sucked in further, and the obstruction will increase. You will note that the child will be struggling to breathe and in distress.

You must go to hospital. Please call 999 and ask for an ambulance now.

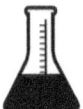

CIRCULAR ITCHY RASH

This is often a roundish rash with reddish color, which may point to a fungus like candida (Thrush), allergies (nettle rash), urticaria (hives) or insect bites.

The borders are often raised, and may not be itchy.

Common causes of this symptom are dry skin, eczema, psoriasis, and meningitis.

Rashes on the palm of the hands, on the feet and on/in the mouth can be caused by viruses and sexually transmitted diseases.

Please do not borrow others' creams or apply steroid cream and/or Vaseline without a proper diagnosis, because these can help a fungus to grow and spread all over your body. Antiseptic washes can also kill helpful bacteria living on our skin and help fungi grow faster.

Keep the affected area well ventilated and dry.

Use a cream or special shampoo as recommended by your pharmacist.

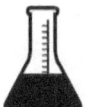

CIRCULAR NON-ITCHY RASH

Ring worm (Tinea) can affect many parts of the body, in particular the groin and scalp. It is most noticeable on bare skin, where it is referred to as ringworm due to its characteristic appearance as a circular patch of red, itchy skin, which gradually increases in size.

There may also be red itchy areas around the base of hair shafts. With scratching, these areas can bleed and become crusted with blood.

This is not a worm, simply a fungus (Tinea).

Prevention: Keep the area well ventilated and dry. Use a separate face cloth and towel. Do not borrow from or give yours to other people. Ringworm is infectious.

Possible complications: Bacterial infection from scratching the affected area is common.

Keep the area well ventilated and dry. Use a cream or special shampoo as recommended by your pharmacist.

Do not borrow others' creams or use steroid cream and/or Vaseline without a proper diagnosis. This can help the fungus grow. Antiseptic washes can also kill helpful bacteria living on our skin and help the fungus grow faster.

You must consult a chemist and get an antifungal cream like miconazol or canistin (often used for athletes' foot and thrush). This rash is contagious and can spread to others.

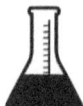 COLD

The cold is the most commonly occurring illness in the entire world, with more than 1 billion colds per year reported in the United States alone.

The common cold is a self-limiting illness caused by any one of more than 200 viruses. The common cold produces mild symptoms usually lasting only 5–10 days. In contrast, the flu (influenza), which is caused by a different class of virus, can have severe symptoms.

A cold is not a disease, but a word used to describe a combination of symptoms that has no treatment, e.g., a runny nose, fever, bodily pain, and coughing. To stop abusing antibiotics, the doctors must start making the correct diagnosis of rhinitis, tonsillitis, pharyngitis, sinusitis, pneumonias or atypical pneumonia, and prescribe the right antibiotics, not broad-spectrum antibiotics.

Flu is caused by one virus called the influenza virus, but there is no treatment to cure this infection.

Some authors of medical textbooks have listed the "Common cold" as an infection caused by various viruses. In the past, this word was probably used to describe Asthma (Chronic Obstructive Lung Disease).

Please consult doctors to get the right diagnosis and treatment.

Please do not abuse antibiotics. It is not good for you to take them unnecessarily, because your body will then become colonized with antibiotic resistant bacteria.

If you have recurrent coughs and colds, it is likely you are suffering because you are allergic to something, or are an undiagnosed asthmatic.

Please choose three symptoms that you have, and follow the instructions as described below.

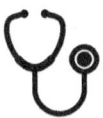 ## COLD AND SHIVERING

This is not a symptom that is associated with the common cold, flu, or a runny nose. This is often seen in patients after surgery, labor or after any invasive procedure.

This is also defined as chills and rigors or feeling hot and cold. This symptom is often associated with serious infections that can rapidly get worse and kill.

It is likely that the infection is in the blood stream, and may result in septicaemia. Serious common bacterial infections (urinary tract, pneumonia, appendicitis, meningitis and glomerulonephritis) all present with mild fever.

This is a common symptom that is often associated with bacterial infections that can rapidly get worse. You must consult a doctor and get the correct diagnosis and antibiotic.

Unfortunately, emerging viral infections like Ebola are also mimicking this symptom and confusing doctors.

The majority of patients will require hospitalization, IV fluids and IV antibiotics. You may require a high dose of antibiotics, so that the amount entering the blood stream will be high enough to kill the bacteria. If low dose antibiotics are prescribed, the bacteria will hide or develop resistance.

Please choose the associated symptoms that you are experiencing. If you do not have any associated symptoms, it is unlikely to be due to a medical illness, and may be environmental in its source.

Please do not rush to a hospital or clinic without speaking to your doctor, because this is one of the symptoms that occur early on if you have the Ebola viral infection.

It is important to let the doctor know your symptoms before visiting a healthcare center. Infections are spread by contact, so you may catch another infection, or pass on yours to doctors, nurses and other patients.

Please consult another doctor if you feel the doctors or nurses are not listening to you. In thirty years, I have seen too many patients become critically ill because the nurses or GPs have reassured them and treated this symptom as a viral infection or prescribed low dose antibiotics.

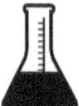 COLD SORE

This is a virus which lives in nerve endings in the skin. It makes its presence felt around the corners of the mouth with crusty, oozing blisters.

A tingling, itchy feeling is usually felt just before the rash forms. Tiny blisters then appear, usually at the lips, where they join the skin. The blisters become sore and itchy. They then crust over, and last about one week before disappearing. They can return at any time.

This condition can be gained by kissing someone infected with herpes simplex. The virus is infectious, particularly when the blister is erupting.

There is not much you can do to prevent catching a cold sore other than avoiding kissing people who have obvious signs of it on their face. Once infected, avoid sudden changes in temperature and sun exposure.

Potential complications: there is a related form of herpes which can infect the genitals, and which can be transmitted through oral sex.

Use simple painkillers such as Paracetamol.

Use a lip salve with a high sun protection factor (SPF) before going into bright sunlight.

Acyclovir cream (e.g., Zovirax) will limit the outbreak if started as early as possible. Ask your pharmacist for advice.

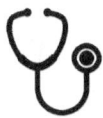 ## CONFUSION

The most common cause of this symptom may be infection, metabolic conditions like diabetes, chemical poisoning, or neurological problems. The problem is how to differentiate between bacterial and viral infections.

This may be how some parents, partners, carers of the children or elderly explain delirium, describing the affected person as talking funny or confused.

This is a common symptom in the elderly and children with acute viral infections, and is associated with very high fever.

It is also seen in elderly patients who have dementia, have a long-term illness, or occult infection like a urinary tract infection, pneumonia, and some viral infections.

The diagnosis of this symptom requires proper clinical examination and may require investigation.

The most common type of infection in the elderly is urinary infections.

Doctors will only treat this symptom after ruling out serious illness, so please consult a DOCTOR and not a nurse in the UK.

Please do not panic, but go to A&E if you cannot get an appointment or you cannot speak to or consult a doctor.

First try to find out why, and for how long, the patient has been confused. Diagnosis of this depends on age and the existence or not of the following symptoms:

- Acute confusion – May be anxious or agitated.
- The presence or absence of hallucinations.
- Variability of performance and/or mood.
- Patient is distant, or experiencing recent memory loss, and/or confabulation.

Common causes are: an infection, especially respiratory and urinary tract infections, an irregular heartbeat, Arrhythmia, Low blood pressure, a heart attack – Painless myocardial infarction, strokes and transient ischemic attacks (TIA), drugs – especially anti-parkinsonism drugs, alcohol, digoxin, sedatives, urinary retention, pain, dehydration, and constipation with faecal impaction.

Less common causes include anaemia, diabetes, uraemia, hypothermia, hypo or hyperthyroidism, Vitamin B12 deficiency, or a head injury.

Social isolation, deafness and blindness can contribute.

Please do not panic, but go to A&E or the ER if you cannot get an appointment or you cannot speak to or consult a doctor.

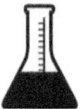 ## CONJUNCTIVITIS

A sign of infection that presents with sticky discharge from one or both eyes.

An allergic reaction may present as watering plus itching only.

This is also called red eye, pinkeye (in the USA) and madras eye (in India).

This is an inflammation of the conjunctiva – the outermost layer of the eye – and of the inner surface of the eyelids.

This commonly occurs when dust, allergens, irritants or a foreign body enters the eyes. Bacterial or viral infection is just one of the causes, but need not be the one and the only cause that requires treatment.

Bacterial infections are commonly unilateral (affecting one eye), and will spread to other eyes if they are not adequately treated.

Bilateral conjunctivitis is more common in viral infections.

Conjunctivitis is said to be an early symptom seen in patients suffering from an Ebola infection.

Bacterial conjunctivitis must be treated with chloramphenicol eye drops every two hours, plus ointment at night for 4–5 days until cleared.

Please perform lachrymal massage after you use eye drops, and continue treatment for 48 hours after the eye looks normal.

Opticrom, and Rhynochrome drops are the treatment of choice for allergic conjunctivitis.

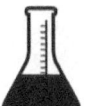

CONTACT LENS STUCK IN EYE

This is a common problem that can be distressing and occasionally painful.

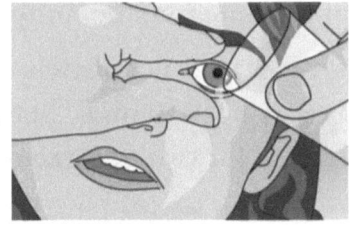

If you are using contact lenses on a regular basis, you may have encountered this problem. Once the contact lens gets stuck, it is often difficult to remove.

Infections and dehydration can result in low tear production, making the lenses get stuck to the sclera.

Treatment is using plain water to wash the lenses.

Please do not use a finger and remove the lens by force.

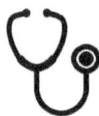 ## CONVULSIONS

"Fits" is a common word used to explain fainting, epilepsy and convulsions.

Convulsions typically have three stages: acute rigidity, loss of consciousness, and a generalized tonic and clonic stage (stiffness and relaxation), resulting in a shaking episode and subsequent drifting to sleep.

Parents get anxious when their child develops high fever, because fits are associated with fever.

Fits occur when the body temperature increases rapidly (suddenly).

Most mothers of children who were brought to hospital with fits felt guilty when we told them the fever was the cause of the fits.

The reason they could not identify this was because the body temperature rapidly increased, precipitating a fit. It is difficult to prevent fits associated with fever.

If you have identified fever in a child, please follow the instructions in the notes and do not panic.

Please do not distress a febrile child just to record the temperature as it is not essential, but make sure you give them paracetamol or junifen for two to three days.

In the case of fits/convulsions, make sure that the patient is breathing, and feel the pulse rate. Do not try to put any object into the mouth. Fits will continue for a few minutes and they will then enter a relaxed state. Please go to hospital, or call 999, because convulsions can occur again.

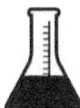 ## CORNS AND CALLUSES

A hard, thickened area of skin is called a callus. A corn is a thickened area on the skin due to friction rub – constant pressure applied on one area. Corns and calluses form on the feet and can make walking painful.

Corns are hard, small patches of thickened skin which often present on the tops and sides of the toes. There are hard, soft, thin and seed corns.

Calluses are hard, rough areas of skin that can develop on hands, feet, or anywhere there is repeated friction.

There are numerous types of corns and calluses, but the treatment is all the same.

Feet if moist and sweaty can breed fungal and bacterial infections. Staph (bacterial) infections can start when bacteria enter corns through breaks in the skin and cause the infected skin to discharge fluid or pus. If you cut a corn or callus and cause it to bleed, the break in the skin invites infection.

If a corn discharges pus or clear fluid that means it may be infected or ulcerated. Both conditions require prompt medical attention.

If you are diabetic, a transplant patient, on steroids, or immunosuppressed, please consult a doctor.

Warts are a hard lump caused by a splinter or foreign body. Warts are viral, and often cause black dots in the affected skin. They also require specific treatment.

Most calluses are corrected by a variety of measures, including a change in shoes, trimming of the calluses, and sometimes surgery.

Most corns and calluses gradually disappear when the friction or pressure stops.

Podiatrists often shave the top of a callus to reduce the thickness.

Properly positioned corn plasters or pads can help relieve pressure on a corn.

There are also special corn and callus removal liquids and plasters, usually containing salicylic acid, but these are not suitable for everyone.

Oral antibiotics may be necessary if the corn is infected. Any pus must be drained through a small incision.

Moisturizing cream helps soften the skin and remove cracked calluses. The cream must be covered for 30–60 minutes with a plastic bag or a sock.

Gently rub off as much of the callus as you can with a coarse towel or soft brush. Using a pumice stone first to rub off the dead skin from a callus after a bath or shower, and then applying moisturizing cream, can also be effective.

There are also stronger creams containing urea that might be more effective, but do not use these unless they are recommended by your doctor or podiatrist.

Hydrocortisone (steroid) creams, Vaseline, and moisturizing your skin incorrectly can aggravate a fungal condition and should be avoided – especially between the toes.

You may consider surgery to remove a plantar callus, but there are no guarantees that the callus will not come back.

The conservative approach of keeping your feet dry and friction-free helps to prevent corns. Wear properly fitted shoes and cotton socks to reduce skin irritation.

If a podiatrist (a foot specialist), or orthopedic specialist (a bone and joint specialist) thinks your corn or callus is caused by an abnormal foot structure, your walking motion, or hip rotation, orthopedic shoe inserts or surgery to correct foot deformities may help correct the problem.

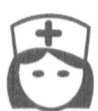 ## COUGH - BARKING TYPE

Coughing is a symptom we all experience from time to time, and most of us will get over them quickly.

There are many different types of cough, and a barking cough is common in children and some adults. Like many symptoms, a barking cough is often not serious in a child, but a cough that sounds sharp – like a bark – can be very distressing.

The commonest cause is a viral infection, croup (acute trachea-bronchitis) which means the trachea and bronchus are inflamed.

At home, being kept well hydrated will help the child. Also, although there is no real evidence that it works, inhaling moist air does seem to help some children, and you can try that to make them more comfortable. However, if at any point the child appears to be having trouble breathing, you should get them to a doctor as soon as you can.

This symptom often occurs in the early hours of the morning (3–4 am), and is often frightening for parents. This is said to occur because there is a dip in atmospheric pressure at this time, and all respiratory problems get worse.

Doctors do not have any special treatment for this, but will act to prevent dehydration, give analgesics, and observe the patient until they get better. Some children may be treated with inhaled steroids (large doses) to suppress inflammation in the larynx (throat area).

In an adult, a barking cough is an indication that there is swelling in the upper part of the respiratory tract, similar to pharyngitis. This can also occur in children, where if the cough is not too severe it may not be croup.

With children or adults, if you have any doubt you should see the doctor.

As with any complaint that happens suddenly and is not accompanied by a cold, a barking cough should be monitored carefully.

If the cough is accompanied by coughing up blood, or leads to shortness of breath, the child is not feeding or taking fluids, or has any difficulty in breathing then treat this as an emergency and go to A&E.

 ## COUGH – DRY

This cough is usually dry and spasmodic. It occurs in patients suffering from viral infections, atypical pneumonia, asthma, or allergies

Viruses, allergies and atypical bacteria thicken the walls of the airways and air sacs. This is often called pneumonitis. Oxygen is poorly absorbed via the thickened walls of the alveoli (air sacs in lungs), making you breathless.

The cough may be a wheezy or musical cough of the barking type, but very distressing. You may have incontinence of urine; develop a hernia, or even faint due to exhaustion.

People with postnasal drip or who are smokers often develop a dry cough. The mucus from the sinuses drains down the back of the throat, and the cough caused by this will normally be worse when you lie down, or when you first wake up in the morning.

This is quite common among those who suffer from hay fever, although if an allergy is present that is due to something other than seasonal hay fever, a cough can be present all year round.

Even if you think this is the cause of your morning cough, it is important to have a proper diagnosis made by your doctor.

It is not wise to self-medicate, as many antihistamine preparations will have side effects, and certain type of coughs, like an asthmatic or allergic cough, must not be suppressed.

Nasal anti-allergy spray can help reduce postnasal drip, and asthma inhalers open your airways. The body will then have to get rid of the sputum or phlegm collected in the lungs.

If the dry cough becomes productive, bringing out lots of phlegm after you start using inhalers, please do not take cough mixtures, or think you have an infection and rush back to consult the doctor. The inhalers contain drugs that open the airways, and the coughing reflex is necessary to clear out the secretions that were locked in the alveoli.

Please consult your doctor to get the correct diagnosis and advice on management. Treating this with on and off antibiotics is not in your interest.

 **COUGHING AFTER EXERCISE**

This is a very common symptom that is poorly managed by some doctors and often ignored by patients. A tickly cough, or coughing spasm precipitated by exercise is not normal.

Please consult a doctor and get the right treatment to help prevent or reduce long-term problems and recurrent antibiotic abuse.

Some doctors use the word "Common Cold" to describe a fever, runny nose and cough. We did not find a disease named as a cold in medical literature. Some new editions of medical textbook list the common cold as an illness caused by numerous viral infections. Fever, coughing, and a runny nose are symptoms that can be associated with numerous minor and serious illnesses.

Flu is caused by a viral infection that can be debilitating, but we do not have specific clinical signs to help diagnose it, or drugs to cure this viral infection.

Coughing indicates that your chest is irritated, and there is excessive secretion that the body is trying to cough out.

Some doctors or nurses call this symptom bronchitis – the most common cause of this is an allergy, asthma or due to excessive secretion dripping into your throat from the nose – post nasal drip.

This may also be connected to gastro-oesophageal reflux – acids from the stomach may be entering the chest.

You can use inhalers to prevent this symptom, so please discuss this with your doctor if you feel the problem is not resolved. This is a common problem in children, as parents often do not know or may not have recognized this as a symptom that requires some treatment.

This is not an emergency, but you must consult a doctor.

 ## COUGHING AT NIGHT

Coughing at night or in the early morning may be a symptom that has existed since childhood. If so, the coughs will probably become productive (producing sputum or phlegm) and you may have treated this with antibiotics in the past. It is also possible that taking cough mixtures has become a habit for you. Cough mixtures do not cure this symptom, but often prolong the problem. Please stop buying cough mixtures and consult a doctor. You are likely to be a patient with an undiagnosed allergic cough, asthma or hay fever.

Some patients assume this is an early indicator to warn them that they will soon develop a chest infection, the flu, or catch a cold. Please note that none of these are true.

Patients also consult doctors and demand antibiotics as soon as they have symptoms of rhinitis (a runny nose), because they assume infection in the nose will soon enter the chest and produce a chest infection. This is also not true because although irritants and allergens that irritate nostrils will often irritate airways and lungs at the same time, you would start coughing as soon as the alveoli get filled with fluid that enter (via post nasal drip) your lungs at night.

The best treatment is to use inhalers and see if the symptoms resolve. Once the phlegm is coughed out, the cough stops.

There are not many diseases or cases in medical literature that exist only in the morning or night.

If you are a smoker, then you may be coughing in the morning or at night. This is likely to be productive (coughing out phlegm or sputum). If it becomes persistent, then you should consult a nurse or a doctor. Chronic lung disease or lung cancer may need to be ruled out if you are a smoker, to prevent emphysema (the need for oxygen therapy).

Post Nasal Drip: This is where mucus from the sinuses drains down the back of the throat. The coughing caused by this will normally be worse when you lie down, or when you first wake up in the morning. This is quite common with those who suffer from hay fever, although if an allergy is present that is due to something other than seasonal hay fever, a cough can be present all year round. Even if you think this is the cause of your morning cough it is important to have a proper diagnosis made by your doctor. It is not wise to self-medicate, as many antihistamine preparations will have side effects.

Asthma: People often think that asthma is only about wheezing and having trouble breathing. In fact, sometimes the only indication that asthma is present is a cough at night, or a persistent cough in the mornings, typically a dry cough that does not produce sputum. If this kind of asthma, called cough variant asthma is suspected by your doctor, he or she may ask you to try an asthma inhaler to see if that will help relieve the symptoms.

Gastro-oesophageal Reflux: This condition is caused by acid from the stomach moving back into the throat. It is quite common to experience a morning cough with this condition. See your doctor, who may prescribe antacids.

Medication: Sometimes some of the medicines that we take can cause irritation, and it is a fact that one in five people who take ACE inhibitors report developing a dry cough. If you are taking medication for high blood pressure and have a cough, let your doctor know and he or she may be able to change your medication.

 ## COUGHING EVERY MORNING

Coughing at night or in the early morning may be a symptom that has existed since childhood. If so, the coughs will probably become productive (producing sputum or phlegm) and you may have treated this with antibiotics in the past. It is also possible that taking cough mixtures has become a habit for you. Cough mixtures do not cure this symptom, but often prolong the problem. Please stop buying cough mixtures and consult a doctor. You are likely to be a patient with an undiagnosed allergic cough, asthma or hay fever.

Some patients assume this is an early indicator to warn them that they will soon develop a chest infection, the flu, or catch a cold. Please note that none of these are true.

Patients also consult doctors and demand antibiotics as soon as they have symptoms of rhinitis (a runny nose), because they assume infection in the nose will soon enter the chest and produce a chest infection. This is also not true because although irritants and allergens that irritate nostrils will often irritate airways and lungs at the same time, you would start coughing as soon as the alveoli get filled with fluid that enter (via post nasal drip) your lungs at night.

The best treatment is to use inhalers and see if the symptoms resolve. Once the phlegm is coughed out, the cough stops.

There are not many diseases or cases in medical literature that exist only in the morning or night.

If you are a smoker, then you may be coughing in the morning or at night. This is likely to be productive (coughing out phlegm or sputum). If it becomes persistent, then you should consult a nurse or a doctor. Chronic lung disease or lung cancer may need to be ruled out if you are a smoker, to prevent emphysema (the need for oxygen therapy).

Post Nasal Drip: This is where mucus from the sinuses drains down the back of the throat. The coughing caused by this will normally be worse when you lie down, or when you first wake up in the morning. This is quite common with those who suffer from hay fever, although if an allergy is present that is due to something other than seasonal hay fever, a cough can be present all year round. Even if you think this is the cause of your morning cough it is important to have a proper diagnosis made by your doctor. It is not wise to self-medicate, as many antihistamine preparations will have side effects.

Asthma: People often think that asthma is only about wheezing and having trouble breathing. In fact, sometimes the only indication that asthma is present is a cough at night, or a persistent cough in the mornings, typically a dry cough that does not produce sputum. If this kind of asthma, called cough variant asthma, is suspected by your doctor, he or she may ask you to try an asthma inhaler to see if that will help relieve the symptoms.

Gastro-oesophageal Reflux: This condition is caused by acid from the stomach moving back into the throat. It is quite common to experience a morning cough with this condition. See your doctor, who may prescribe antacids.

Medication: Sometimes some of the medicines that we take can cause irritation, and it is a fact that one in five people who take ACE inhibitors report developing a dry cough. If you are taking medication for high blood pressure and have a cough, let your doctor know and he or she may be able to change your medication.

 ## COUGHING IN ASTHMA

This cough is usually dry, spasmodic and very distressing. It occurs in patients suffering from asthma, hay fever, and other illnesses that produce dry cough.

The cough is typically wheezy, whistling or musical.

People with postnasal drip or who are smokers often develop a dry cough. The mucus from the sinuses drains down the back of the throat, and the cough caused by this will normally be worse when you lie down, or when you first wake up in the morning.

This is quite common among those who suffer from hay fever, although if an allergy is present that is due to something other than seasonal hay fever, a cough can be present all year round.

Even if you think this is the cause of your morning cough, it is important to have a proper diagnosis made by your doctor.

It is not wise to self-medicate, as many antihistamine preparations will have side effects, and certain type of coughs, like an asthmatic or allergic cough, must not be suppressed.

Asthma inhalers open your airways, and the body will have to get rid of the sputum or phlegm collected in the lungs. If the dry cough becomes productive – bringing out lots of phlegm – please do not take cough mixtures or think you have an infection. Your technique of inhaling drug is likely to be good, and coughing soon after taking this drug indicates that you are responding to the treatment.

If you do not cough more and bring out phlegm or sputum, then please consult your doctor. Your technique may be poor, or you may have an infection that is not allowing the drug to enter the lungs well.

If you are coughing and breathless, use an aero chamber, Volumatic, or spacer to help take the inhaler. Make sure the Volumatic is clean, dry, has been washed using hot water, and has not had a cloth used to dry it. Pump out one or two puffs into the Volumatic, breathe two or three times, and pump again. If you pump more than three times, the amount of the drug entering the chest reduces. The dose used when using a Volumatic must be 3–4 times higher than otherwise. Discuss with an asthma nurse about maintaining the Volumatic, and about how to use this in the case of an emergency.

If you try to take the inhaler directly through the mouth, the drug will stick to your throat and make you develop side effects like vomiting, shaking, palpitations, and feeling as if you are going to have a panic attack.

Please note again that coughing out large amounts of phlegm or sputum after taking the inhaler is good. This is not a sign indicating that you are developing a chest infection. The inhaler drug opens the airways and helps the body cough out the sputum that has accumulated in the alveoli (air sacs).

Do not take any cough mixture or use drugs to suppress the coughing reflex. Using aromatic oils and other irritants will increase nasal secretions and make you cough for a longer time.

If you are not coughing out large amount of phlegm after taking the inhaler, and you are breathless with no audible wheezing, please go to hospital. You may have developed a chest infection, or your technique for using the inhaler is poor.

Please make sure you have the drugs (not expired ones) handy all the time, even if you have not had an asthma attack in the last few years.

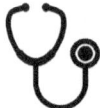 ## COUGHING IN CHILDREN

Coughing is a reflex to prevent dust, allergens, bacteria, or our own secretions entering the lungs.

This is not a disease, nor is it a good initial sign to help doctors diagnose Pneumonia (chest infection) and advise treatment.

Babies often produce a grunt and look as if they are anxious. The grunt occurs because the alveoli (air sacs) of the lungs are filled with thick secretions, leaving no space for oxygen to be absorbed.

Lack of oxygen makes babies develop severe headache and so they become irritable. Crying makes them use more oxygen, and so they are often alert, and look as if they are scared, with wide-open eyes.

This symptom will always be associated with other symptoms, so please check those symptoms too, and act as advised.

The most common cause is postnasal drip. The mucus from the sinuses drains down the back of the throat, and the cough caused by this will normally be worse when they lie down, or when they first wake up in the morning. This is quite common in babies sleeping in overheated rooms with low humidity. Babies can also develop a cough due to allergies, house dust mites, or smells present in the bedroom.

This may be treated with antihistamine preparations, special cough mixtures, and eucalyptus oil sprinkled in the bed. Please do not give cough mixtures or use aromatherapy. This can cause more harm than good.

Parents often think that asthma is only about wheezing and having trouble breathing. In fact, sometimes the only indication that asthma is present is a cough at night or a persistent cough in the mornings, typically a dry cough that does not produce sputum. If this kind of asthma – called cough variant asthma – is suspected by your doctor, he or she may ask you to try an asthma inhaler to see if that will help relieve the symptoms.

Gastro-oesophageal Reflux: This condition is caused by acid from the stomach moving back into the throat. It is quite common to experience a morning cough with this condition. See your doctor, who may prescribe antacids.

Common symptoms associated with this are a sore throat, a runny nose, generalized body pain, sneezing, sweating, a grunt, or being limp and tired.

Please choose one of the following: Dry, wheezy, barking, night, morning, or chesty cough. Also read about Asthma.

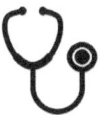 ## COUGHING IN MERS

This cough is often dry, because something known as pneumonitis (walls of the air sacs become thick) develops, and the lungs cannot absorb oxygen, causing air sacs to collapse.

Pneumonia is a general term for an inflammation of the air sacs of the lungs caused by an infection or chemical. With pneumonia, the lungs fill with fluid, which interferes with their ability to transfer oxygen to the blood. MERS is known as an atypical pneumonia, because the usual bacteria and/or viruses do not cause it.

MERS (Middle East Respiratory Syndrome) is a severe, pneumonia-like respiratory disease caused by a virus. It is different from SARS, because MERS is caused by another subtype of the virus.

MERS causes very high fever, unlike normal bacterial pneumonia which develops a mild to moderate fever. It may also produce a cough, and severe shortness of breath associated with dry coughing.

The infection is thought to be spread by close contact with an infected person. A virus called coronavirus is the cause of MERS. There are many kinds of coronavirus, some of which cause the common cold. The MERS coronavirus (MERS-CoV) was a new variant that was discovered in 2012 in the Middle East.

How MERS spreads is not completely understood, but experts believe that the main way it spreads is through close contact with an infected person (by caring for, or living with, the person or having direct contact with their respiratory secretions and body fluids).

The people who have been infected by MERS so far have all been in a health care facility or among close family members.

MERS is different from SARS. Most importantly, the MERS virus does not appear to be as easily spread between people, whereas the SARS virus spreads very easily.

The main symptoms of MERS are: a dry cough, shortness of breath and difficulty breathing, diarrhoea, and high fever (over 38°C or 100.4°F).

PLEASE CONTACT AN ISOLATION HOSPITAL OR CALL THE EMERGENCY MERS HELP LINE. DO NOT GO TO A HOSPITAL OR CLINIC. THE ISOLATION UNIT WILL SEND DOCTORS AND AN AMBULANCE.

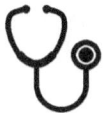# COUGHING OUT BLOOD

A streak of fresh blood on the surface of phlegm or sputum is usually seen if you have a sore throat or a small tear in the pharynx. This is very common but can make you very anxious.

Occasionally, the gums may be bleeding and so the sputum gets coated with streaks of blood.

Streaks of fresh blood in the sputum are not an emergency, but must be discussed with your doctor. If you are young and have had a sore throat or dental problem, please do not panic, but speak to a doctor.

Blood mixed with sputum is called haemoptysis and must be treated as an emergency. Often the blood is not red but dark or black, as the red blood cells get broken down and the iron seeps out.

Common causes are a chest infection (pneumonia), TB, or even a worm infestation.

Smokers must consult their doctor and be referred to specialist care.

If you are coughing out large amounts of red or black blood, please go to hospital, as this is an emergency.

You must consult doctors, preferably a chest physician in the hospital, to get the correct diagnosis after investigations and get the right treatment.

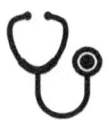# COUGHING OUT FRESH BLOOD

Coughing out fresh blood is called haemoptysis.

This is an early sign of a serious chest infection like pneumonia, TB, and cancer of the lungs, and so must be treated as an emergency.

Smokers must consult and be investigated by a specialist in the hospital.

If you are coughing out large amounts of red or black blood, please go to hospital, as this is an emergency.

You must consult doctors, preferably a chest physician in the hospital, to get the correct diagnosis after investigations and get the right treatment.

Streaks of blood on the surface of phlegm or sputum are common if you have a sore throat or a small tear in the pharynx. This is very common, but can make you very anxious. This is not an emergency, but you must consult a doctor.

If you are young and have had a sore throat or dental problem, please do not panic, but speak to a doctor.

Occasionally the gums may be bleeding, and so the sputum is coated with streaks of blood.

If bleeding has occurred in the lung, the blood is not red but dark or black, as the red blood cells get broken down and the iron seeps out.

Common causes are a chest infection (pneumonia), TB, or even a worm infestation.

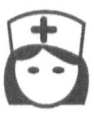 ## COUGHING OUT GREEN PHLEGM

Doctors used to diagnose infection and prescribe antibiotics once the patient produced green phlegm or sputum. In 1990, it was proved not to be associated with infection, so doctors do not now give much importance to the color of sputum.

To diagnose the cause of this symptom, doctors will ask about other associated symptoms.

Treating this as a chest infection using low dose antibiotics is not safe, because the dose of antibiotics entering the chest is very low and so can help bacteria develop resistance, create an antibioma (abscess), or make good bacteria living in our body develop resistance.

Some doctors will send sputum for culture, and check which antibiotics work. This is useful but not always necessary. We anticipate this to become routine practice if the trend of spreading antibiotic resistant bacteria in the community becomes very common.

If your doctor has diagnosed this as an infection, and prescribed antibiotics, but you are not getting better, please go back and ask the doctor to refer you to hospital care. Antibiotics prescribed at the right dose will kill sensitive bacteria, and you should be getting better after taking them three times in twenty-four hours. If you are not better, you may be infected with resistant bacteria or virus.

Please speak to, or consult a doctor.

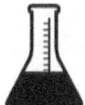

CRADLE CAP

Seborrhoea dermatitis in infants presents as cradle cap.

A thick white or yellow waxy scale builds up on the scalp.

There is no bleeding or obvious irritation unless too vigorous attempts are made to remove it.

There is no fever and the child is perfectly well.

Routine cleaning will prevent it in most cases.

There are no serious complications.

Cradle cap clears up in a few months. A form of eczema, it responds well to simply rubbing the affected parts of the scalp with olive oil. Leave it on overnight before washing it off with a mild shampoo in the morning. Like many other forms of eczema, the cause of cradle cap is unknown.

Shampoos are available from your pharmacist but you should try rubbing with olive oil first. If it is severe, try low dose sulphur and salicylic acid cream, applied at night. Ask your pharmacist for advice.

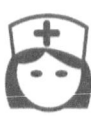 ## CROUPY COUGH

This is a common symptom of a night illness in children. The cough starts off with a load stridor (noisy breathing), and must be distinguished from the two other causes of stridor: epiglottitis, and an inhaled foreign body

Please do not open the mouth, check the temperature orally, or make a child with stridor cry – this may precipitate complete airway obstruction.

If acute stridor developed when the child was eating or playing, or developed suddenly with no other signs of illness, think of an inhaled foreign body.

There are many different types of cough, and a barking cough is one that is associated with croup. This is common in children and can be quite alarming.

The commonest cause is a viral infection called croup (acute trachea-bronchitis), meaning that the trachea and bronchus are inflamed.

Symptoms often occur in the early hours of the morning (3–4 am) and are often frightening for parents.

In an adult, a croupy or barking cough is an indication that there is swelling in the upper part of the respiratory tract, similar to pharyngitis. This can also occur in children, where if the cough is not too severe it may not be croup.

With children or adults, if you have any doubt you should see the doctor.

Keep the child in a comfortable position and do not get over anxious, as this will make the child more anxious.

Treatment of croup is steam inhalation, sitting the child in a bathroom full of steam or boiling a kettle in the bedroom. Steam inhalation is not proved to be of benefit, but is harmless. Some parents say it helps, and so it is worth trying.

Make sure the child is comfortable and not crying – the child is irritable because of anoxia (oxygen supply to brain is low), and will have a headache. Place the child in a comfortable position (in the arm of the mother or on a bed – let the child decide).

If the cough is accompanied by coughing up blood, or leads to shortness of breath or any difficulty in breathing, then treat this as an emergency and go to A&E.

At home, being kept well hydrated will help the child, and although there is no real evidence that it works, inhaling moist air does seem to help some children, and you can try that to make them more comfortable. However, if at any point the child appears to be having trouble breathing, you should get them to a doctor as soon as you can.

Doctors do not have special treatment, but will prevent dehydration, give analgesics, and observe the child until they get better. Some children may be treated with inhaled steroids (large doses) to suppress inflammation in the larynx (throat area).

Treat this as an emergency and go to hospital if you or the child is cyanosed, restless or drowsy.

If the child is looking very anxious, has a fast heartbeat, intercostal recession, and has continuous stridor, please call an Ambulance and your doctor.

 # CRYING BABY

The common causes of a baby's crying are hunger, thirst, a wet nappy, constipation, a urinary infection. An acute ear infection, sore throat, urinary tract infection, foreign body, obstruction to airway, pneumonia, gastro-enteritis (tummy pain) and torsion testis, volvulus, intestinal obstruction, and a strangulated hernia are some of the common causes of excessive crying.

Babies often develop a headache if they have difficulty breathing. This is common when a child has croup or blocked nostrils

Some children with syndromes may have an irritable cry.

People assume that pulling the leg up and crying is associated with the baby having tummy pain. This is not 100% true, but some babies with urine infections and/or constipation do have tummy pain.

Babies unable to drink milk or eat food because of an infection in the mouth like thrush, or a sore throat can also cry a lot.

Bottle fed babies will struggle to breastfeed because they have to suck harder than from the bottle.

If the baby is drifting to sleep when breast-feeding, please make sure the baby has sucked well. Babies struggling to feed often suck in air that fills the stomach with wind. These babies wake up in the middle of the night, or a couple of hours after their feed, and start crying.

Hungry babies may not wake up and cry, because their blood sugar goes low. This is neuro-hypoglycemia, and is very common. If the baby does not wake up to feed, please wake them up and feed them every two or three hours.

Pain in the ear due to wax or infections also causes babies to cry, but this symptom is also associated with other symptoms. The most common causes are hunger, a wet nappy, separation anxiety, or colic.

Doctors do not know what causes colic. But we have noticed that babies with poor feeding technique cry. The most common cause of this is air phage, i.e., sucking in air when feeding. This happens when the teat or bottle has a small hole. Babies get tired, open their mouths in between feeds, and swallow air. Trapped wind will stretch the stomach and produce a rumbling noise that may be painful.

This can also happen when the mouth is not properly latched on to the nipple of the breast.

Using Portex disposable bags and feeding bottles will help reduce aero phage. Some doctors, chemists and nurses will recommend drops or powders to use. These may or may not help, but are worth trying. If the baby pulls its legs up, the baby may be constipated or have a urinary tract infection.

Please check the associated symptoms before rushing to hospital.

Please note that some babies (more boys than girls) develop projectile vomiting because they have developed tightening of the stomach (pyloric stenosis), and these babies are often very hungry.

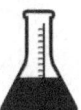 **CRYING BABY DURING FLYING**

This is a very common problem that is distressing to parents and annoying to other passengers. Parents struggle to console the baby, and find it especially hard because the problem occurs during take-off and landing.

This problem occurs because the pressure in the middle ear of the baby increases, producing excruciating pain. If the baby has symptoms like blocked nostrils or an ear infection, the pressure can burst open the baby's ear drum resulting in a perforated ear drum.

Please consult a doctor and get nasal drops, (ephedrine or xylometazoline nasal drops). You must use the drops thirty minutes to an hour before take-off and also before landing if you are on a long haul flight. This will keep the Eustachian tube open, so that middle ear pain does not occur.

Make sure you have a bottle with milk ready, or use a dummy so that the baby can start sucking during take-off and landing. If you do not have both, just put your finger in the baby's mouth and make them suckle. This prevents blockages in the ears, and should stop babies experiencing pain.

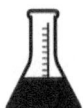

CYSTITIS

Women suffer most from this infection of the bladder, which makes you pass water more often, and may cause it to sting when you do. Men appear to get off lightly because of the greater distance between the anus, from which most of the bacteria come, and the urethra, through which urine is passed.

The most common causes to rule out are a bacterial infection, kidney stones, or diabetes.

Preventative measures include drinking plenty of fluids and going to the toilet to empty your bladder more often.

Put a covered hot water bottle against your tummy to ease the pain.

Drink slightly acidic drinks such as cranberry juice, lemon squash, or pure orange juice. Try a mixture of potassium citrate available from your pharmacist.

If the treatment given by the chemist has not helped, and you still feel infected after 6–8 hours, or if there is any blood in your urine, please consult a doctor.

If you are pregnant, take a urine sample from your first visit to the toilet in the morning to the practice nurse. Use a clean, well-rinsed bottle.

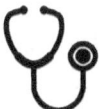

DELIRIOUS

This is a common symptom that is associated with very high fever. People often describe this as "talking funny" or "nobody can understand what he or she is saying."

This problem is often associated with viral infections, but doctors find it hard to be 100% certain this is a viral infection because some metabolic disorders can also produce this symptom.

Diagnosis of this symptom is often not easy, and requires proper clinical examination and sometimes investigation. Experienced doctors will only treat this symptom after ruling out serious illness so please consult a DOCTOR.

Please do not panic but go to A&E or the ER if you cannot get an appointment or speak to a doctor.

The most common causes of this symptom are an infection, a metabolic condition like diabetes, chemical poisoning, or neurological problems.

The problem is to differentiate between bacterial and viral infections. The diagnosis of this symptom requires proper clinical examination and may require investigation.

This may be how some parents, partners, carers of the children or elderly may explain delirium by describing the affected person as talking funny or confused.

This is a common symptom in the elderly and children with acute viral infections, and is associated with very high fever.

It is also seen in elderly patients who have dementia, have a long-term illness, or occult infection like a urinary tract infection, pneumonia, and some viral infections.

Doctors must clinically examine and investigate to rule out infections and other causes of behavioral changes.

The common causes are a urinary infection, diabetes, dehydration, metabolic disorders, alcohol, the effects of prescription drugs, and drug abuse.

Doctors will only treat this symptom after ruling out serious illnesses.

Please do not panic but go to A&E or the ER if you cannot get an appointment. IF you are finding it hard to take the person to hospital or a clinic, call 999.

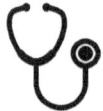 ## DIABETES

Please refer to Disclaimer. If you are diabetic, or looking for information to advise others with diabetes, please STOP. Do not use MAYA.

Diabetes, often referred to by doctors as diabetes mellitus, describes a group of metabolic diseases in which the person has high blood glucose (blood sugar), either because insulin production is inadequate, or because the body's cells do not respond properly to insulin, or both. Patients with high blood sugar will typically experience polyuria (frequent urination), and will become increasingly thirsty (polydipsia) and hungry (polyphagia).

Diabetes is a long-term condition that causes high blood sugar levels. In type 1 diabetes the body does not produce insulin. 10% of all diabetes cases are said to be type 1. In type 2 diabetes the body does not produce enough insulin for proper functioning. 90% of all cases of diabetes worldwide are of this type. Gestational Diabetes can affect females during pregnancy.

The most common diabetes symptoms include frequent urination, intense thirst and hunger, weight gain, unusual weight loss, fatigue, cuts and bruises that do not heal, male erectile dysfunction, numbness, and tingling in hands and feet.

If you have Type 1 and follow a healthy eating plan, do adequate exercise, and take insulin, you can lead a normal life.

Type 2 patients need to eat healthily, be physically active, and test their blood glucose. They may also need to take oral medication, and/or insulin to control blood glucose levels.

As the risk of cardiovascular disease is much higher for a diabetic, it is crucial that blood pressure and cholesterol levels are monitored regularly.

As smoking might have a serious effect on cardiovascular health, diabetics should stop smoking.

Hypoglycaemia – low blood glucose – can have a bad effect on the patient. Hyperglycaemias – when blood glucose is too high – can also have a bad effect on the patient.

Please consult your doctor.

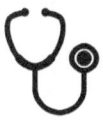 ## DIARRHOEA IN MERS

MERS (Middle East Respiratory Syndrome) is a severe pneumonia-like respiratory disease caused by a virus. It is different from SARS because MERS is caused by another subtype of the virus.

MERS is known as an atypical pneumonia, because the usual bacteria and/or viruses do not cause it. The walls of the air sacs in the lungs are thickened, reducing oxygen supply to the other organs.

The people who have been infected by MERS have all been in a health care facility or among close family members.

MERS is different from SARS. Most importantly, the MERS virus does not appear to be as easily spread between people, whereas the SARS virus spreads very easily. The main symptoms of MERS are: coughing, shortness of breath, and difficulty breathing. Diarrhoea and a high fever (over 38°C or 100.4°F) is also one of the presenting symptoms. PLEASE CONTACT AN ISOLATION HOSPITAL OR CALL THE EMERGENCY MERS HELP LINE. DO NOT GO TO A HOSPITAL OR CLINIC. THE ISOLATION UNIT WILL SEND DOCTORS AND AN AMBULANCE

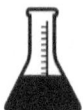

DIARRHOEA WATERY

This is a common symptom that is often managed poorly because nurses and doctors have been giving conflicting opinions, and naming this as tummy flu, gastro-enteritis, tummy bug, tummy upset and even as gastritis.

Watery diarrhoea occurring within 6 hours after eating some food or drink is often due to chemical irritation, and unlikely to be an infection.

The patient is likely to be vomiting, so may have tummy pain due to increased intestinal motility. The best treatment is NOT TO DRINK PLAIN WATER, but to drink water with dioralyte or electrolyte powder in it for 24 hours.

Please note that the intestinal wall cannot absorb water or food during this time, so YOU MUST NOT EAT OR DRINK FIZZY DRINKS OR SOLIDS.

Solid food is first liquefied in the stomach, then nutrients are absorbed through the intestinal wall. When the tummy is sick, the wall cannot absorb any nutrients other than plain water, but requires one molecule of salt and one molecule of glucose to do so. This is known as facilitated absorption.

If kids do not drink fluid, or hate dioralyte, the best drink is some NON-FIZZY COLA. Please add two to three PINCHES of salt to every glass or can of coke. You need this salt to help water absorption, and it will also help to reduce fizz. Some mothers have been silly and not followed this advice due to worrying about their children's teeth. The result of this callous act resulted in these children getting severe dehydration and almost dying in hospital.

Please do not try to make your own electrolyte solution by adding salt and sugar to water. We have encountered serious problems because the salt intake was too high, resulting in a condition called hypernatremia dehydration which can be fatal.

If the symptom is associated with other symptoms, or there is blood and mucus in the stool, please check "dysentery" or "stool with blood and mucus" and follow the advice there.

It is important to know, that dehydration and anaemia are major problems that result in kidney and liver failure. Please start rehydration using electrolytes mixed with water.

If diarrhoea is associated with other symptoms, or there is blood and mucus in the stool, please consult a doctor.

Typhoid and cholera can start as watery diarrhoea and get worse within hours. Please note that the bacteria that cause these infections have rapidly become resistant to treatment. The only option you have is to avoid contact with the infection and eating contaminated food. This common illness will be a major problem in countries where there are too many houseflies and poor sanitation.

If you are living in a place where the Ebola viral infection is endemic and spreading, please speak to a doctor before rushing to clinic or hospital. The reason you must not rush to hospital is to help protect you from getting infections from other patients visiting clinics or hospitals.

85% of patients with the Ebola viral infection presented with diarrhoea. We are also trying to reduce infection spreading in the community and to healthcare workers. Doctors can use video consultation linked to the MAYA App, and offer help and advice to help you get better.

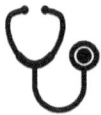 DIARRHOEA WITH BLOOD

Fresh bloodstains on the toilet roll used to clean your anus is not caused by dysentery, because the stool will be black or tarry (black) colored if the bleeding is in the intestine.

Blood that you may have occasionally noticed dripping into the pan is often due to fissures and tears in the anal area. Constipation, anal sex, or trauma can produce tears in the anal region.

This common problem causes people to panic and rush to hospital.

If the watery stool contains blood and mucus, this is called "dysentery." This is often due to a worm infestation, amoebiasis, or problems in the intestine.

If the diarrhoea is associated with a fever, this may be typhoid. Check the patient's temperature. If it is high and the heart rate is low – and not high as generally seen in various infections – please ask your doctor to rule out typhoid.

You may have developed a rose colored rash, and if a blood test is positive, you will need special drugs and hospital care.

You must contact a tropical disease specialist for advice and treatment.

Amoebic dysentery and other intestinal infestations must be investigated.

Please consult, and get investigations, if a tear or fissure is noticed in the anus.

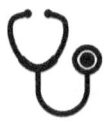 ## DIARRHOEA AFTER RETURNING FROM HOLIDAY

Please note that dysentery is the name used to describe diarrhoea containing blood and often mucus. This is a common infection in various tropical countries and so must be investigated. This is often due to a worm infestation, amoebiasis, or a problem in the intestine.

This is a common problem seen in patients returning from a holiday. If the watery stool contains blood and mucus, please treat this symptom as "blood in stool."

If the diarrhoea is associated with fever, this may be typhoid. Check the patient's temperature. If it is high and the heart rate is low – and not high as generally seen in various infections – please ask your doctor to rule out typhoid. You may have developed a rose colored rash, and if a blood test is positive, you will need special drugs and hospital care.

You must contact a tropical disease specialist for advice and treatment.

Amoebic dysentery and other intestinal infestations must be investigated. A stool check and blood test must be done to find the cause.

If you are returning from an Ebola infected area, please speak to a doctor before visiting a clinic, surgery or hospital.

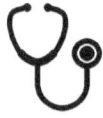

DIARRHOEA IN EBOLA ENDEMIC AREA

85% of patients with Ebola virus infection presented with diarrhoea.

It is important to know that dehydration is a major problem that results in kidney and liver failure. Please start rehydration using electrolytes mixed with water but do not drink plain water.

If you are living in an area where the Ebola viral infection is endemic and spreading, please speak to a doctor before rushing to a clinic or hospital. The reason you must not rush to hospital is to help protect you from getting infections from other patients admitted to or visiting clinics or hospitals.

We are also trying to reduce infection spreading in the community and to healthcare workers. Doctors can use video consultation and also offer help and advice to help you get better.

YOU MUST NOT EAT OR DRINK FIZZY DRINKS OR SOLIDS FOR 24 HOURS. The tummy is sick and cannot absorb any food because it lacks enzymes to digest food.

If kids will not drink the prescribed fluids, the best drink is some NON-FIZZY COKE. If you add two or three pinches of salt to every glass of coke, it will lose its fizz and also work like an electrolyte solution.

Please do not try to make your own electrolyte solution with salt and sugar. We have encountered serious problems before, because the salt intake was too high, resulting in a condition called hypernatremia dehydration which can be fatal.

If this symptom is associated with other symptoms, or there is blood and mucus in the stool, please check "dysentery" or "stool with blood and mucus," and follow the advice there.

Please do not leave home, but make sure you call the help line and get the hospital isolation unit to send an ambulance to pick you up and organize isolation.

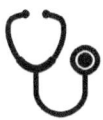 DIFFICULT TO BREATHE

You need to be more specific about the problem. This is a phrase often used by patients but, doctors cannot understand this wording.

Are you breathing fast, slowly, irregularly, or are you choking?

Doctors or nurses must not offer advice via telephone for this, and must insist on clinical examination.

If this symptom is associated with severe chest pain lasting more than 15 minutes, vomiting, or pain radiating to the jaw or arms, please call an ambulance and go to hospital.

Sudden onset of breathlessness is not a common symptom, and must always be treated as a medical emergency.

Chest infections caused by bacteria often present with a mild to moderate fever, followed by breathlessness and no cough. The right name of this chest infection is "Pneumonia," and it must be treated as an emergency.

Oral antibiotics are not the right treatment to start. You will need intra-venous antibiotics given in large doses. Antibiotics given by mouth are poorly absorbed, so will only kill good bacteria and provide an opportunity for resistant bacteria to grow.

Anxiety attacks, panic, and stress can also make some people complain of catching breaths or air hunger, and they will often have associated symptoms like palpitations (audible heart sounds), tachycardia (increased heart rate), or a tingling sensation in their fingers and/or toes.

If the symptom is acute and you feel dizzy, please call 999 and ask for an ambulance to take you to hospital. Please do not drive.

Asthma, chest infections, aspiration, and acidosis are some of the common conditions that cause breathlessness. These are illnesses that can only be managed in hospital.

This symptom is often associated with other red symptoms, but please treat this as an emergency and consult a doctor even if this happens to be the only red symptom. Please go to A&E or the ER.

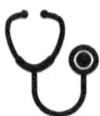 ## DYSARTHRIA

Dysarthria means having difficulty speaking because there is a lack of coordination of the facial muscles due to a neurological deficit.

Is not a common symptom, but is often associated with vertigo, head injuries, alcohol intoxication, neurological problems, drugs, and infections.

There are numerous causes and so this is very difficult to diagnose. This will require specialist help.

Please consult doctors now, or go to a hospital.

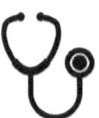 ## DISCHARGE FROM PENIS OR VAGINS

If you notice white discharge from your penis after unprotected sex, then you must consult a doctor in the GUM (Genital-Urinary Medicine) or STD (Sexually Transmitted Disease) Clinic in the hospital.

In the UK, you do not require an appointment, but can walk in and get tests and treatment.

PLEASE NOTE THAT THIS IS CONFIDENTIAL, so no one other than the doctor and you will know what disease you have.

He or she will not inform your doctors if you let them know that you do not want this.

You will also get tested for other sexually transmitted diseases. It is important to know that the symptoms may resolve without treatment, but you will still risk spreading the infection to others and may develop complications later.

Common sexually transmitted bacteria that are spreading in the UK and USA are said to have rapidly become resistant to treatment.

Diseases like gonorrhoea, syphilis, and chlamydia are becoming very difficult to treat, so please go to a GUM or STD clinic as soon as possible.

Gonorrhoea is a common sexually transmitted disease and so easily passed between people through; unprotected vaginal, oral or anal sex, sharing sex toys that haven't been washed or covered with a new condom each time they're used. The age of patients is between 15–24 years.

Super Gonorrhoes is rapidly spreading al over the world and is difficult to treat or control.

Typical symptoms of gonorrhoea include a thick green or yellow discharge from the vagina or penis, pain when urinating and (in women) bleeding between periods. One in 10 infected men and almost half of infected women don't experience any symptoms.

Gonorrhoea is usually treated with a single antibiotic injection and a single antibiotic tablet. With effective treatment, most of your symptoms should improve within a few days. You must attend a follow-up appointment a week or two after treatment, so another test can be carried out to see if you're clear of infection.

You must avoid having sex until you've been given the all-clear.

PLEASE CONSULT A DOCTOR IN A GUM CLINIC

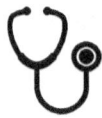 **DISMENNORHOEA**

This is pain associated with menstruation (periods), and its common name is period pain.

The most common cause is hormonal changes, but this can also be associated with infections, fibroid uterus, or abnormalities in other endocrine glands like the thyroid or pituitary.

Period pain is often associated with excessive bleeding.

If you are sexually active, and had unprotected sex, please get a pregnancy test.

If bleeding is profuse and you are passing clots, you may need to go to hospital and consult a gynaecologist.

If you are a teenager or a young girl who has recently started having periods, this may be hormonal change.

Paediatricians must see any pre-pubertal girl with bleeding and pain, because this could be traumatic and the child may develop psychological problems in the future.

Please consult a doctor and go to a GUM or STD clinic if you had unprotected sex with a new partner and then developed this symptom.

If you are not sexually active, please consult a chemist and start taking a Non-Steroidal Anti-inflammatory drug (mefenemic acid, brufen) a day or two before your period is due. This helps to regulate your hormones, prevent pain, and reduce blood loss. If you are suffering from gastritis, or ulcers in your stomach, please consult a doctor instead, and do not take NSAID.

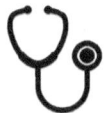 # DIZZINESS

The cause of dizziness in adults and elderly is often vertigo. This occurs because the nerve in the ears responsible to maintain our balance is affected.

Feeling dizzy can be very annoying and worrying, but is probably not serious.

If the feeling of dizziness persists, you should certainly be checked out by a doctor.

Feeling dizzy may leave you feeling off balance or lightheaded, or you may feel that everything around you is spinning.

This symptom can be acute or chronic. If acute, this is sudden onset dizziness (first time feeling this way), and means you need urgent consultation. If this is chronic, i.e., has happened before, do not panic, but start treatment as for the previous time(s).

The main causes of dizziness in adults and elderly are drugs, ear problems, and vertigo.

Doctor will rule out serious illnesses, and may give anti-sickness pills or antihistamines to reduce the swelling of nerves in the ear.

You may be advised to use steam inhalation, followed by the nasal spray Beconase (Beclomethasone) or Pulmicort (Budesonide) to decongest the sinuses of children and young adults with chronic dizziness.

Serc is a drug often used, but you must be on this treatment for a few weeks.

The diagnosis of this symptom requires proper clinical examination and may require investigation.

Doctors will first check blood pressure, so you must consult as soon as possible.

Shingles in the ear can produce dizziness because the nerve in the ears swells up.

If this symptom is associated with other red symptoms, you must go to hospital now.

If dizziness occurs when you get up out of bed, or stand up from a sitting position, you must speak to a doctor and get your blood pressure and drug treatment reviewed.

If the dizziness that you suffer is sudden, very debilitating, or associated with blurred vision, you must see a doctor.

Please do not drive to hospital but call an ambulance to take you.

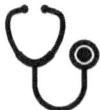 DOG BITE

Make sure the doctors are aware if the main purpose of the visit is to document your injuries for a possible future compensation claim. Ask doctors to record the details carefully.

First, you need to determine that the animal was a dog, fox, cat or other type of animal.

It is best to take a picture of the bite mark when it is fresh, so that the doctor can see and document the bite marks.

If fresh, there will be a reddish area surrounding the wound. This is called as Cellulitis.

If the wound is old and infected, you will notice discharge, and may have other associated symptoms can that help you identify a serious problem. You must treat this as an emergency, because infection can spread through the blood and result in septicemia.

Doctors will perform blood tests, take a wound swab for culture and check sensitivity.

Management is to irrigate (if a fresh wound).

Ask about prophylactic antibiotics in the case of: Complicated dog bites affecting the hand or genital area, moderate or severe injury, crushing injury, oedema, and/or the wound penetrating bone or joints.

Discuss with your doctors if you are immune-compromised, diabetic, on steroids, or the wound is near a prosthetic joint.

Keep infected arms or legs elevated.

Consider the need for vaccination against tetanus and post-exposure prophylaxis against rabies.

Consult a doctor, or go to A&E.

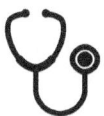

DOUBLE VISION

This is currently not a common symptom, and must be seen in the eye clinic of a hospital.

Occasionally you may have double vision when you are about to faint, have a fit, go into septic shock, are dehydrated, or your blood sugar drops (Hypoglycaemia). In these cases you will have other associated symptoms that can help us diagnose the cause.

Please do not waste time trying to identify the cause using the Internet.

Please go to a walk-in eye clinic, or speak to your doctor

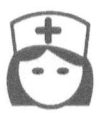

DRINKING MORE WATER

Diabetes is the most common cause, if this symptom is associated with excessive thirst.

If you are forcing yourself to drink excess water because someone told you to drink more water every day, then the problem is likely to be what we call psychogenic polyuria and polydipsia.

You can get a blood sugar test done in a local pharmacist. If the sugar level is high, make an appointment to consult a nurse.

If you have other associated symptoms like vomiting, weakness, or loss of weight, please treat this as an emergency.

The other potential cause, though rare, is a kidney and endocrinal (hormonal) problem.

This is an acute problem that requires an emergency appointment. If you are vomiting and/or have other symptoms like weight loss, you must go to hospital.

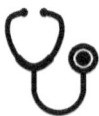 DROWSINESS

The first things that doctors will think of in this case are low blood sugar, dehydration, depression, lack of sleep, and types of exhaustion like burnout.

This may be a symptom associated with an environmental (e.g., excessively hot or cold weather), metabolic (salt and water abnormality, dehydration, low sugar) or endocrinal (diabetic, hypothyroidism and others) problem.

When levels of salt and sugars go down in your body, you will be drowsy, because the body has an inbuilt mechanism to slow down its metabolism to conserve energy.

The brain needs constant flow of sugar because it is working 24/7, 365 days a year. Low blood sugar will produce a condition known as neuro-hypoglycaemia, that makes you drowsy. When you experience this, you will realize that it is hard to think, and should get some food to eat and so boost the sugar level in your body.

Babies who have difficulty feeding, have diarrhoea and are vomiting will often be drowsy because their body has low sugar levels.

Try drinking high calorie drinks, or eating some chocolate and see if you feel better.

Dehydration is also a common cause, but please remember that you need sugar and salt to help water absorption and so YOU MUST DRINK DIORALYTE (Read about "diarrhoea" and "vomiting").

Severe infections that result in septicemia can also make you drowsy, because the bacteria are consuming your food and water.

Consult doctors if this problem is on-going.

If acute, please go to a hospital and speak to a doctor.

Please note that 39,000 people die in the UK every year because the nurses and doctors in primary care fail to identify septicemia early. We think that there are millions of people dying because they do not give adequate importance to this symptom.

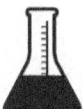
DRY EYE

This is a common symptom in the elderly, because they produce less tears and the eye becomes dry.

Inflammation of the cornea due to allergies, an infection, or trauma can result in dry eyes.

This is often associated with various drugs, mixed connective tissue disorders, rheumatoid arthritis, ulcerativEtis, thyroid problems, and numerous illnesses seen in the elderly.

The herpes simplex virus is an infective cause, the corneal ulcer being diagnosed by testing with fluorescein.

You need a specialist to deal with this problem, because dry eye(s) will be one of the symptoms of generalized illness.

Doctors will often request various blood tests, and may perform visual tests to rule out serious problems in the eyes and make the right diagnosis.

Please consult a doctor, because damage to the cornea such as ulcers can be prevented if treated early.

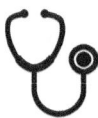 ## DRY MOUTH

This symptom is commonly experienced during the night or when waking up in the morning. This symptom refers to a sticky, dry feeling in the mouth, often accompanied by frequent thirst, sores in the mouth, sores or split skin at the corners of the mouth, and/or cracked lips. You may also experience a burning or tingling sensation in the mouth and especially on the tongue, a dry, red, raw tongue, hoarseness, dry nasal passages, problems speaking, or problems tasting, chewing or swallowing.

This is not a common symptom and you must be seen by a doctor.

This is a known side effect of drugs such as antidepressants, beta-blockers, antihistamines, diuretics, bronchodilators, steroid inhalers, and blood pressure treatments. It may also be connected to dehydration, fever, sweating, blood loss or burns. It is associated with diseases and infections like, Sogren's syndrome, diabetes, anaemia, cystic fibrosis, rheumatoid arthritis, hypertension, stroke, Parkinson's disease, mumps, and damage to the salivary glands due to radiation or chemotherapy.

A damaged nerve in the neck can cause this.

Tobacco and alcohol use may contribute to this symptom.

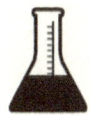 **DRY SKIN**

Excessive washing of the hands and body can often dry skin out.

Dry, itchy skin is common in the elderly, and may get infected.

You may be an asthmatic – please discuss this possibility with your doctors and get the right treatment. Please note that you can develop symptoms of asthma even if you are old.

This is not an illness that you are always born with, but can be associated with allergies. An allergy is an exaggerated reflex, designed to help protect us from potentially toxic substances that would make us ill. Please remember that things can go wrong in our body at any time of life.

The usual treatment of this symptom is emollients and creams that can be bought in the chemist. Doctors do not have special drugs to treat this, so please ask a chemist to help.

The majority of doctors are generously prescribing steroid creams for this. This quick-fix solution is not one that good doctors will offer. We have seen dermatologists generously prescribing steroids as a first-line treatment. They claim it is based on evidence based medicine, but this we feel is wrong because these drugs can cause long-term problems.

Please note that steroids are not drugs that can cure any disease or illness. This is like covering up muck using a carpet. Inflammation is suppressed, reducing redness and stopping the itching. Prolonged or regular use will suppress your immunity, and so you will become prone to infections that may increase morbidity and mortality.

Please consult a doctor if the dry skin is cracked, bleeding or has started secreting turbid, or yellowish fluid.

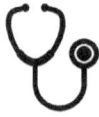
DYSENTERY

Diarrhoea with blood and often mucus in it is called "Dysentery."

This is a common infection in various tropical countries, and must be investigated. It is often due to a worm infestation, amoebiasis, or problems in the intestine.

If the diarrhoea is associated with fever, this may be typhoid. Check the patient's temperature. If it is high and the heart rate is low – and not high as generally seen in infections – please ask the doctor to rule out typhoid.

You may have developed a rose colored rash, and if a blood test is positive, you will need special drugs and hospital care.

You must contact a tropical disease specialist for advice and treatment.

Amoebic dysentery and other intestinal infestations must be investigated.

Fresh bloodstain on the toilet roll used to clean your anus is not caused by dysentery, because the stool will be black or tarry (black) colored if the bleeding is in the intestine.

Blood that you may have occasionally noticed dripping into the pan is often due to fissures and/or tears in the anal area.

Constipation, anal sex or trauma can produce tears in the anal region. Please consult a doctor, and get investigations if a tear or fissure is noticed in the anus.

If you are returning from an Ebola infected area, please speak to a doctor before visiting a clinic, surgery or hospital.

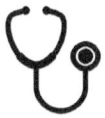 # DYSPHAGIA

This is an inability to swallow solids or liquids.

Patients can present with saliva dribbling out of their mouth, and being unable to swallow. This is common in patients with facial palsy or strokes, and in children with epiglottitis (check stridor). In most cases it is quite painful, and its most common presentation is sore throat that is presented with difficulty in swallowing and loss of voice.

This is a common symptom when the throat is inflamed, red and painful. This is inflammation of throat, and not swollen tonsils.

Patients find it hard to swallow, and have difficulty talking because of the inflamed upper part of oesophagus.

Like many types of inflammation, pharyngitis is characterized by a rapid onset and is typically a relatively short lived symptom.

Pharyngitis can result in very large tonsils, which cause trouble swallowing and breathing.

Pharyngitis may be accompanied by a cough (which can be painful), and fever.

Most acute cases are caused by viral infections, with the remainder caused by bacterial infections, fungal infections, or irritants such as pollutants or chemicals.

Treatment is mainly symptomatic, although bacterial or fungal causes may be treated with antibiotic or anti-viral medicines respectively.

This is a very early and common symptom seen in 57% of patients with Ebola, and this is now called Ebola Odynophagia or dysphagia.

Patients report or complain of pain while swallowing.

This pain while swallowing can be described as an ache, burning sensation, or occasionally a stabbing pain that radiates to the back of the throat.

Minor and serious problems, such as abnormalities in the oesophagus must be ruled out before doctors can offer advice or treatment.

Foreign bodies can also cause obstructions and result in this symptom.

A damaged oesophagus or a fungal infection can make swallowing difficult.

Patients on large doses of steroids or cytotoxins, and who are immunosuppressed, or organ transplant patients can present with this symptom.

Patients with blood disorders and serious illness like discriminated intravascular coagulation (DIC) can present with a sore throat and inability to swallow. This is an emergency, and so must be referred to and managed in hospital.

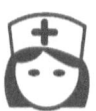 ## DYSUREA

The most common cause of burning sensation when passing urine in adults and children is a urinary tract infection.

Women often assume that this symptom is cystitis, and try to fight the symptom by drinking water, Cranbury juice or electrolyte powders that help change the pH of urine to make it less irritating to vaginal mucosa.

Unfortunately, antibiotic resistant bacteria that do not respond to treatment now threaten us. Reducing delay in establishing the diagnosis and getting treatment early is essential. Please make an appointment with the nurse and get your urine checked early to help reduce future complications.

Please make sure you get your blood pressure checked regularly.

Babies and children may start vomiting or cry when passing urine. Children often develop constipation because they are afraid to pass urine. They may also have associated symptoms (like fever, increased frequency of urination or anuria) to help confirm the diagnosis.

To confirm the diagnosis you will need a urine culture and microscopy. If blood and proteins are present in urine, the nitrate test is often positive. But if the infection is tested for early, this test may be negative. Please note that this test does not always confirm or rule out the presence of infection, and so must not be relied upon. Patients have developed serious septicaemia because they did not receive the right treatment early.

Please do not waste time before starting treatment if you have all the symptoms that suggest a urinary tract infection, but please make sure you have collected and sent a sample of urine off for testing (microscope and culture sensitivity) in the laboratory.

E.Coli is a common cause of this symptom, and we know the majority of its organisms are resistant to treatment. It has become very difficult to manage these common infections.

If symptoms like fever, and pain when passing urine are not better after taking three doses of antibiotics, please consult your doctor and do not go back to the nurses clinic or a walk-in-clinic.

You must check the lab results before changing the antibiotics or getting admitted to hospital for intra-venous antibiotic treatment.

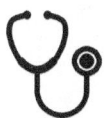

EAR WITH WATERY DISCHARGE

This is rare, but is often seen after head injury with a crack in the base of the skull. Cerebro-spinal fluid drains out from the meninges through the nose or ears.

Using a dipstick (used to check urine) will show if the fluid has sugar in it.

This is an emergency, and you must be seen by doctors in hospital.

Melting wax (seen if you develop ear infection) is usually turbid and drains out from the ear even before you start feeling unwell, or develop a fever or ear pain.

If the discharge is foul smelling, and the ear canal is itchy, you may have an infection in the ear canal which can be treated with eardrops.

Please do not pack your ears with cotton or try to clear the discharge using ear buds, because you may introduce an infection or impact the melting wax.

Please consult a nurse if there has been no fall or indication of an injury to the head.

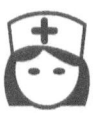 **ECZEMA**

This presents as areas of dry flaky skin, most often on the flexor (skin) surface over the elbow and knee. It is more common in young people and old people.

The term dermatitis means exactly the same thing, but tends to be used when the eczema is caused by contact with a chemical or other irritating substance.

Atopic eczema is an allergic condition and runs in families.

People who suffer from other allergies such as hay fever are also more prone to eczema.

The dry flaky skin is often worse in winter, but can also occur throughout the year.

Contact dermatitis can be very severe, with the skin becoming deeply inflamed, leading to skin loss. The underlying deep skin looks red and angry. Secondary infection is common because of the itching.

Seborrhoea dermatitis is the name for eczema that affects the scalp and eyebrows. A thick, yellow, greasy scale builds up, leading to heavy dandruff.

Atopic eczema is probably an inherited condition. This inflammation flares up as a response to an allergy, although the source may never be identified. Hair dye, nickel watch-backs, jewellery and washing powders are all known to cause contact dermatitis in susceptible people. If you identify the precipitating factor, you can avoid those substances, materials or chemicals and cure yourself.

This may be a fungal infection, although it could equally be an extreme form of allergy affecting the hairy parts of the body.

Please note that eczema can occur because of emotional stress. Children can develop eczema when they change home, start school or experience separation anxiety.

You must keep the skin moist using emollient ointments. Your pharmacist will advise you on this.

Use a bath water additive, which contains moisturizing oils.

Secondary infection may occur, particularly in very young children.

Unfortunately using topical steroid creams, which can so effectively suppress symptoms of eczema, is becoming a major problem for doctors to prescribe. This quick-fix solution is not one that good doctors will offer. We have seen dermatologists generously prescribing steroids as the first-line treatment. They claim it is based on evidence based medicine, but this we feel is wrong because these drugs can cause long-term problems.

Please note that steroids are not drugs that can cure any disease or illness. This is like covering up muck using a carpet. Inflammation is suppressed, reducing redness and stopping the itching. Prolonged or regular use will suppress your immunity, and so you will become prone to infections that may increase morbidity and mortality.

Please consult a doctor if the dry skin is cracked, bleeding or has started secreting turbid, or yellowish fluid.

There exists a wide range of products which will help stop the itchiness and keep the skin moist.

Scratching and itchiness can be reduced by keeping the skin moist and taking antihistamine tablets or medicine. This is useful for young children, as it also has a mild sedative effect, making for a better night's sleep for everyone.

Speak to your doctor if the eczema is spreading very quickly, or the skin is becoming infected or painful.

Use cotton, linen and gloves or mittens at night to prevent scratching.

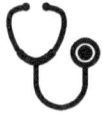 EYE HARD

Pain in the eye is often very severe and may be associated with vomiting. This symptom refers to a hard and tender eye, with gross reduction of vision. This may be preceded by sub-acute attacks which cause haloes to appear around lights.

This is an emergency – sight can be lost within hours.

You will require eye drops every few minutes to try and constrict the pupil and reduce pressure in the eye while awaiting the ophthalmologist.

Please go to hospital now.

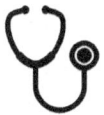 # EYE IS RED

Red eye can be very alarming; if you feel as if the eye is gritty when you open and close the eye, it is not usually a sign of anything very serious. More commonly, it will be a sign that you have conjunctivitis or another type of minor eye problem.

Usually the redness is not painful but if it is, this might be a sign of something a bit more serious.

If there is acute pain with the redness, and the eye is not sticky, then you should go hospital.

You should see a doctor in the eye clinic in hospital if the red eye is associated with the following:

Your eyes are sensitive to light, your vision is reduced, you are feeling sick (or vomiting), you have a severe headache, or your vision is blurred.

While conjunctivitis is the most likely cause of a painless red eye, the next most likely reason for the red eye without pain is a blood vessel that has burst. You must get your blood pressure checked in this case.

Conjunctivitis is the swelling and irritation of the conjunctiva. The conjunctiva is the thin layer of tissue that covers the eyeball and the inner surfaces of the eye. If this layer gets swollen, the eye will look bloodshot, and it may feel as though there is grit in it.

An irritant like dust or chlorine from a swimming pool can cause conjunctivitis, and it might also be due to an allergy or an infection.

Conjunctivitis that is due to an allergy will normally affect both eyes and be very itchy.

Viral conjunctivitis, on the other hand will usually affect one eye first, making it water, and then will show as redness in the other eye a few days later.

Viral conjunctivitis is quite often seen with the common cold.

Although a red eye is not normally an indication of anything serious, it is always a good idea to see the doctor if the condition persists, or if you have pain with the redness.

The majority of patients we see in surgery are the ones who stopped their treatment early, used eye drops only 2–3 times every day, or did not perform lachrymal massage.

Please note that eye drops must be used once every 2–3 hours in both eyes and should be accompanied by massage of the lachrymal gland. Please watch a video on YouTube to see how to massage your lachrymal gland to prevent re-infection.

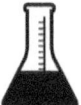 **EYE ITCHY**

Most of us will, at one time or another have suffered from itchy eyes. The eyes might also be puffy and red. Although this is not usually very serious, it can be very irritating.

It is a fact that although having itchy eyes is very common, most people do not really know what causes it. The most common cause of itchy eyes is allergic conjunctivitis.

Along with the itchiness, there will probably also be problems with the throat, the nose, and possibly even the head as well.

If the itchy eyes are experienced mostly in the spring, the time that allergies often affect hay fever sufferers, or if you know that you have been exposed to something that you are allergic to, then it is pretty obvious what is causing the itching.

Many people and some doctors label this as a common cold and sinus infection. Some virus infections can make the eyes very itchy and red, but in that case you will also have fever at the same time.

Since the symptoms are very similar to an allergy, it is important to properly differentiate and offer the right diagnosis and treatment.

If you are not sure, you can wait a few days to see if the symptoms subside as the cold does, or note if you have other symptoms such as sneezing and a sore throat before you go to the doctors.

If you think that you are suffering from conjunctivitis (itchy eyes accompanied by redness and a wet or sticky discharge around the eyes), you should speak to a chemist for advice.

Conjunctivitis is contagious, especially among children. Please make sure the child stays at home until the symptoms subside. Some mothers are sending their children to nursery or school when they are infected because they cannot afford to pay a baby sitter or have someone come to take care of their children. This must be discouraged, because the bacteria that cause this infection are resistant to treatment. By sending your child to school, you can actually pass on infection to another child (who may be immune-suppressed or on steroids) who might catch this infection and die.

Blepharitis (allergic rash on the eyelid), can also cause itching of the eyes. Along with the itching you may also notice that there is redness and swelling of the eyelids as well as flakes in the eyelashes. If you think that you have blepharitis, you should make an appointment to see the doctor.

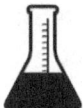 **EYE STICKY**

This common symptom of the eyes is caused by infection. There are some substances like smoke, gases, smog and pollen that can also produce inflammation that looks as if it is an infection. This is easy to diagnose and start treatment.

If you are using eye drops – PLEASE use the drops once every 2–3 hours for 1–2 days, then start using cream four times daily.

You must use the drops in both eyes, otherwise infection from one eye will move to the healthy eye.

YOU MUST DO LACHRYMAL MASSAGE - Please find information on this via Google. If you do not do this massage, the infection will come back. Do not use contact lenses when on treatment for this.

Please read "Eye itchy," "Eye red," "Eye pain" and "Eyes are watery" for more information.

Consult a doctor if you are a mother with a sexually transmitted disease (HIV, Gonococcus or Herpes) and have a new-born baby with sticky eyes.

 **EYELID HAS A LUMP**

This is more likely to be a sty if it is associated with pain.

This small painful lump appears on the edge of the eyelid and gradually become bigger.

Chemists will provide an ointment that must be used four times every day for five days.

Eye drops are not useful, because they are diluted by tears. Bacteria need to be killed by a large dose of antibiotics.

Using ointment helps, but it must be used 4 times every day. You must also make sure you massage the lachrymal gland (Please use the Internet to check how to do this).

If styes are occurring regularly, please consult a doctor and find out why.

Using hot water can help to ease the pain, and helps the sty to open and discharge its secretions.

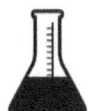 EYES ARE WATERY

This is a very common symptom associated with Hay Fever, exposure to some allergenic substance or smoke, or occurring when you are emotional.

You must first try self-treat before consulting a doctor, because doctors will first offer the same treatment that a chemist would advise.

A common treatment is anti-allergy eye drops that block allergens from attacking the eyes. Unfortunately, you have to use the drops twice every day for six weeks.

You must also use a nasal spray to help reduce sinus congestion. Tears are drained through the nose, so mucous membrane inside your nose will swell up and produce a blocked nose. These blocked nostrils will prevent tears coming out, and so you will experience excessive tears rolling out from the eyes.

Please note that this drug will only work for 12–24 hours and not cure your illness. If the problem is chronic, please do not assume you have a recurrent cold.

Read all about allergic conjunctivitis and blepharitis, and make sure you get the correct treatment.

Please note that there is no drug that cures this, but only those that offer symptomatic treatment – symptoms will stop only while you use the eye drops.

Babies with this symptom have blocked tear ducts. Learn how to massage the tear ducts situated near the base of the nostrils, and make sure you perform lachrymal massage.

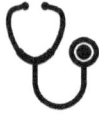 ## EYES LOOK YELLOW

Having a yellow tinge to the whites of the eyes is often a sign that you have a mild attack of jaundice.

If you have canary yellow tinged eyes, please consult a doctor because this could be an early sign of anaemia that requires vitamins B12 and folic acid. This is often a missed or neglected symptom. Please read about pernicious anaemia. If treated properly with vitamin injections on a regular basis, you will not develop long-term complications.

If the whites of your eyes are very yellow, then it is quite likely that your skin will also be yellow (look at the tip of the nose).

Jaundice is quite common in new-borns, but it can affect people at any age, and be variable in its intensity. If an affected baby is not feeding well, and is drowsy and lethargic, please consult a doctor because the baby may develop long-term problems. Please make sure the baby is feeding well, because low sugar will allow jaundice to enter the brain resulting in kernicterus.

Jaundice is what happens when bilirubin builds up in our body tissue and in the blood.

The most common causes for this build-up of bilirubin are a liver condition, such as hepatitis, or the presence of gallstones.

If you have a yellowing of the whites of the eyes as well as a tinge of yellow to your skin, also look at the mucous membranes of the nose and mouth, which may also have taken on a yellow hue. This is cirrhosis of the liver.

When you go to the toilet, you might notice that the urine you pass is darker in color, and that your stools are lighter (whitish) in color.

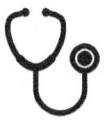 ## EYES PAIN

The most common causes of this symptom are conjunctivitis and glaucoma.

Glaucoma is a medical emergency and will need treatment to reduce the pain and swelling caused by increased pressure in the eyes. This condition will be associated with other symptoms like vomiting, redness, and the eye feeling hard.

Your vision is altered, and you are likely to be an adult. Please note that this can also occur in children but is very rare.

Conjunctivitis is associated with a gritty feeling and sticky eyes. The infection often starts in one eye and spreads to both eyes. The problem is to differentiate between allergic conjunctivitis, bacterial and viral infections, and glaucoma.

The diagnosis of this symptom requires proper clinical examination, and may require investigation.

Doctors will only treat this symptom after ruling out serious illnesses, so please speak to a doctor.

There are numerous causes for this symptom, so you must be seen by an ophthalmologist. You can also call a hospital and ask them if they offer a walk-in eye clinic to deal with emergency eye problems.

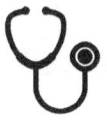 ## EYES WITH FLOATERS

The diagnosis of this symptom requires proper clinical examination and may require investigation.

Doctors will only treat this symptom after ruling out serious illnesses, so please speak to a doctor or consult an ophthalmologist.

There are numerous causes for this symptom, so you must be seen by an ophthalmologist. You can also call a hospital and ask them if they offer a walk-in eye clinic to deal with emergency eye problems.

You must speak to or consult doctors if you have symptoms that are red.

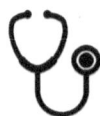
FAINTING

A person who has fainted will not respond to stimuli, but will be breathing (probably shallowly or rapidly), have a palpable pulse (heart beat felt), and may look pale, blue, or feel very hot or cold.

Call 999 and ask for an ambulance.

Check the person's airway, breathing, and pulse frequently. If necessary, begin CPR.

If the person is breathing and lying on their back, and you do not think there is a spinal injury, carefully roll the person towards you onto their side. Bend the top leg so both hip and knee are at right angles. Gently tilt their head back to keep the airway open. If their breathing or pulse stops at any time, roll the person onto their back and begin CPR.

If you think there is a back (spinal) injury, leave the person where you found them (as long as breathing continues). If the person vomits, roll the entire body at once to their side.

Support their neck and back to keep the head and body in the same relative position while you roll them.

Keep the person warm until a doctor or ambulance arrives.

If you see a person fainting, try to prevent a fall. Lay the person flat on the floor, and raise their feet to a level above his or her head. This will help blood circulation to the brain.

Fainting is most likely to be due to low blood sugar. Give the person something sweet to eat or drink when they become conscious.

If the person is unconscious from choking, start CPR. Chest compressions may help dislodge the object from the airway.

If you can't feel a pulse or heartbeat, try a firm bang on the chest using the soft part of your fist (the opposite side to your thumb). This can stimulate the heart if the heart is in shock.

If you see something blocking the airway and it is loose, try to remove it. If the object is lodged in the person's throat, do NOT try to grasp it or forcefully open the mouth. This will push the object farther into the airway.

Continue CPR, and keep checking to see if the object is dislodged until medical help arrives.

DO NOT

- Panic
- Touch the unconscious person without proper inspection of their surroundings (look for live wires, blood, vomit, urine, faeces and saliva).
- Give the person any food or drink.
- Leave the person alone.
- Place a pillow under the head of an unconscious person.
- Slap an unconscious person's face or splash water on their face to try to revive them.

WHEN TO CALL EMERGENCY

If the person is unconscious and:

- Does not return to consciousness quickly (within a minute)
- Has fallen down or been injured, especially if they are bleeding

- Has diabetes
- Has seizures
- Has lost bowel or bladder control
- Is not breathing
- Is pregnant
- Is over the age of 50
- If the person regains consciousness but complains of chest pain, pressure, or discomfort, or has a pounding or irregular heartbeat
- If the person cannot speak, has vision problems, or cannot move their arms and legs

Prevention

To prevent becoming unconscious or fainting:

- Avoid situations where your blood sugar gets too low.
- Avoid standing in one place too long without moving, especially if you are prone to fainting.
- Drink lots of fluids (preferably flat coke with pinch of salt – see dehydration treatment), particularly in warm weather.
- If you feel like you are about to faint, lie down, or sit with your head bent forward between your knees.
- If you have a medical condition such as diabetes, wear a medical alert necklace or bracelet.
- Please Read: "Unconsciousness," "Altered state of mind."

 **FALL**

You must consult a doctor if your legs, hand, wrist or any other part of the body is swollen and painful.

Doctors will often clinically examine you, check your blood pressure, and request investigations like blood tests and scans.

Please check your associated symptoms using MAYA if you have any other symptoms

Always think of any drugs you are on that may be causing this symptom.

Common causes are Parkinson's disease, drugs (especially over sedation), postural hypotension (low blood pressure) including that which is drug-induced, immobility, (e.g., that due to rheumatoid or osteoarthritis), muscle wasting or connective tissue disorders, cardiovascular causes, (arrhythmias), fits, drops attacks, vertigo, Meniere's disease (Shingles in ears), TIAs,, and strokes.

Metabolic causes include diabetes, anaemia, low potassium, dehydration (low fluids), and hypothyroidism.

Confusion associated with this symptom may be connected to a urinary infection in the elderly.

Please go to hospital if you have severe bleeding, or have other symptoms that are colored red.

If you are an elderly person, such people often fall because they have fractured their hip. Please do not expect doctors to visit you at home and offer any treatment other than painkillers. Doctors will often request an X-Ray to rule out fractures, so please go to your local A&E or ER.

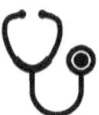

FATIGUE

This is a vague symptom and you must be very specific. Do you feel tired after performing physical tasks, generally tired, feel low and want to sleep, or do you have weakness in your legs or arms?

Interpretation of this symptom is difficult because fatigue can be associated with depression, drug abuse, infections, and metabolic and endocrine problems.

This can also occur due to deficiencies or a neuromuscular disorder.

In the past ten years, there have been numerous patients with fatigue diagnosed as having ME. This condition is associated with various viral infections, and so can be difficult to diagnose.

We have seen some patients respond to antidepressants, but management of this condition in this manner is very controversial.

Please consult your doctor, and maybe get a referral to consult a neurologist or a psychiatrist.

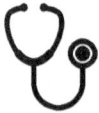 FEELING COLD

This may be because you are exposed to a cold climate, have reduced peripheral circulation (dehydration, septic shock), or have a hormonal problem.

Feeling cold and shivering, known as chills and rigors, is often associated with infections that can rapidly get worse. This symptom associated with infection is more serious than a high or very high temperature.

You must consult a doctor and get the correct diagnosis and antibiotics. It is likely the infection is in the blood stream and so may result in septicaemia, shock and death.

Unfortunately, emerging virus infections are also mimicking this symptom. The majority of patients will require hospitalization and IV antibiotics.

You may require a high dose of antibiotic so that the amount entering the blood stream is high enough to kill the bacteria. Bacteria or toxins released into the blood by bacteria are called septicaemia or blood poisoning.

Please note, antibiotic resistant bacteria have more enzymes and toxins than the meningococcal infection that produces meningitis. The resistant bacteria and emerging viruses can produce numerous organ failures, which make it very difficult to resuscitate, and to manage the condition. Please read all about Antibiotic Resistance in this book and be prepared.

Doctors must not prescribe low dose antibiotics if they are sure the symptom has occurred due to infection. Bacteria will hide from low doses, develop resistance, become more virulent, and spread in the community.

Please choose the associated symptoms that exist. If you do not have any associated symptoms, this is unlikely to be due to medical illness, and may be environmental.

Please go to a hospital and consult a doctor as an emergency if the associated symptoms are all red.

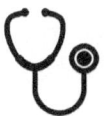 FEELING HOT AND COLD

The symptom is also called Chills and Rigors. Feeling hot and cold is often associated with infections that can rapidly get worse.

You must consult a doctor and get the correct diagnosis and antibiotics.

It's likely that the infection is in the blood stream, and so may result in septicaemia. Serious common bacterial infections (urinary tract infection, pneumonia, appendicitis, meningitis and glomerulonephritis) all present with mild fever, as can septicaemia.

At times, you may have a very high fever, suggestive of viral infection. The temperature will soon change to feeling hot and cold. This is very suggestive of secondary bacterial infection.

Unfortunately, emerging viral infections are also mimicking this symptom.

Majority of patients will require hospitalization and IV antibiotics. You may require a high dose of antibiotic so that the amount entering the blood stream is high enough to kill the bacteria.

If low dose antibiotics are prescribed the bacteria will hide or develop resistance. Your temperature and symptoms should reduce after taking three doses of the correct level of antibiotics, if the symptoms are not reduced, tell your doctor.

Malaria is one of the infections in tropical countries presenting with this symptom.

Please consult another doctor if you feel the doctors or nurses are not listening to you. In thirty years, I have seen too many patients become critically ill because the nurses or GPs have reassured them and either treated this as a viral infection or prescribed low dose antibiotics.

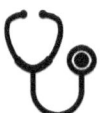 **FEELING LOW**

This is a common problem doctors encounter. They will find it hard to differentiate between feeling weak or lethargic, and burnout, stress, or depression.

It is important for you to be specific. If you are not, the doctors will refer you to a psychiatrist, and soon your condition will be labeled as depression and you will be put on pills like Prozac.

I have seen too many people suffer because they are on pills they don't need, and have a poor quality of life because the drugs are chemicals that interfere with the thought process.

If you are low, first you should try to understand yourself. Find out why you feel low – speak to your partner or parents, but not friends. Get help from the right people.

Personal coaches, NLP and videos published by various people are available on the Internet to help you. The best adviser will often be a stranger, because they do not know you personally or have any hidden agenda.

Please go through these before you visit a doctor, and do not expect medical professionals to have a magic pill to cure your illness.

You will also find questionnaires on the Internet to help you identify the cause.

Think hard before being labeled as having depression and becoming hooked on to pills for the rest of your life.

I have always said that psychiatric illness is one that we can cure provided we listen well and identify the cause. If you are finding it hard to sleep because your mind is constantly thinking of the problems you have at work, then you will feel low.

Sleep, oxygen, food and water are the only essential things to sustain life. Lack of sleep will make you feel low and depressed.

I discourage you from seeking help from doctors if you are feeling low.

In 2005, I did a pilot study to see why some patients aged 50 years old have big bundles of notes where others have one card in their file. I was surprised to see 100% of these patients with large amounts of notes had only psychiatric illnesses.

When I looked at what happened when they were children, I noticed that their parents had consulted doctors 13–26 times in a year. It was obvious to me; the mother was depressed, and so visited the doctor complaining about her child (Munchausen's by proxy).

The GP had failed to identify that the problem existed in the mother and not the child. This child had grown up, and as an adult remembered rushing to doctors whenever they are sick, and so lost confidence and became dependent on doctors. It's easy to identify these patients as doctors. When I ask them, "What do you think is wrong with you?" the answer is always the same "You are the doctors. You know, not me."

The doctors who see this child as an adult rushing to consult with trivial problems will label them as a hypochondriac. He or she will be referred to a psychiatrist and labeled as having mild, moderate or severe depression. They will soon be popping pills, and become dependent on counselors, clinical psychologists and psychiatrists.

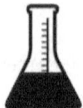 **FEVER**

Please note that the presence or absence of fever is a very important sign and symptom that helps doctors to differentiate common from serious illnesses.

Please choose the right type of fever (no fever, mild, moderate, high, very high, feeling hot and cold, or chills and rigors) to help MAYA to advise you.

We have listed "No Fever" as an option because two symptoms in a person with no fever are as important as having three symptoms. E.g., If you are breathless, coughing and feeling hot and cold, then the cause of the illness could be bacterial or viral pneumonias, but if you are not feeling hot and cold (no fever) then the diagnosis is more likely to be asthma, a panic attack, chemicals or drugs.

If you ask a doctor for advice because you or your child have a high fever, the doctor will not be able to diagnose the problem or offer advice and offer treatment based on this alone. They will ask numerous questions to find out why you have a fever, so please go through the types of fevers in MAYA.

Fever is also known as pyrexia, and is a common medical sign characterized by an elevation of the body temperature above normal levels.

Fever on its own does not help doctors diagnose any illness. Normal body temperature can increase in healthy adults and children after 30 minutes of activity or exercise, anxiety, or excitement, and 1 hour after eating food. Sexual excitement (blushing) also increases your body temperature, breathing, and heart rate.

Infection is one of the things that can result in increased body temperature.

Antibiotics can only kill the bacteria, but do not help to reduce the body temperature. 98.6°F was established as Normal in 1868, but this has been muddled since (Jama 268: 1578–78, 1992).

If the body temperature increases every day, please book an appointment to consult a doctor.

In certain infections, fever is beneficial because bacteria will die when the body temperature increases. Gonococci and Syphilis are killed when the body temperature increases above 40°C. A high temperature can also reduce nutrient absorption and stop bacteria from multiplying. Moderate fever also accelerates the immune response and so helps us kill the bacteria

Most bacterial infections that produce serious illness like meningococcus, pneumococcus, and some viruses produce enzymes that help them control the thermoregulatory center in the hypothalamus (brain).

Please note that parents, family, nurses, and receptionists often give more importance to a child with a high fever than an adult with mild or moderate fever. We do not know how people were made to believe this, because an adult (above 12 years old) with mild fever is in a more serious condition than a child with high fever.

We have always followed this rule (and at times annoyed nurses and some parents in the hospital) to prioritize a teenager or young adult with mild or moderate fever.

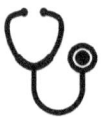 **FEVER AND FITS**

This is known as febrile convulsions. It affects 3–4% of children, chiefly between the ages of 1–5 years, often those with a family history of febrile fits.

Please note, infection is one of the causes that result in increased body temperature. Antibiotics can only kill the bacteria but does not help to reduce the body temperature or prevent fits.

Do not get anxious when a child has a high temperature, because fits occur when the temperature has gone up rapidly. If you identify fever, then the body temperature is raising slowly. You can start treatment and prevent fits.

In the last thirty years of medical practice, we have never seen one child develop fits because the body temperature was very high.

Most mothers of children who were brought to hospital with fits felt guilty when we told them that the fever was the cause of the fits.

The reason they could not identify this was because the body temperature rapidly increased, precipitating a fit. It is difficult to prevent fits associated with fever.

If you have identified fever in a child, please follow the instructions listed below and do not panic.

Please do not distress a febrile child just to record the temperature as it is not essential, but make sure you give them paracetamol or junifen for two to three days.

Please follow the instructions listed below and do not waste time calling doctors or rushing to hospital without giving the treatment of lukewarm water bath to help reduce temperature.

The main task is to identify the precipitating cause, like tonsillitis, otitis media, urinary tract infections (UTI), and to rule out meningitis.

Please read about fever and types of fever and be safe.

If the child or you must go to hospital, please call an ambulance because fits can occur again.

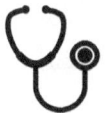 ## FEVER IS MODERATE

The most common cause of this symptom is likely to be infection. Bacteria do not thrive in very hot or cold environments but viruses do. A moderate temperature creates ideal conditions for bacteria to live and multiply.

This is a simple and logical way to help differentiate between bacterial and viral infections.

The diagnosis of this symptom requires proper clinical examination and may require investigations like blood tests and scans.

Doctors will only treat this symptom after ruling out serious illnesses, so please consult a DOCTOR. Please do not panic, but go to A&E or the ER if you cannot get an appointment, or you cannot speak to or consult a doctor.

 # FEVER Temp 36-38°C or 98-100°F

Some parents are keen and believe the reading on a thermometer is very important. To tell you frankly, I have not given any importance to this recording since graduating as a doctor, knowing that it can vary every five minutes depending on the body's metabolic rate, activity and whether a child is in distress (crying).

When we have a mild or moderate fever, we assume that we have a mild illness or mild virus infection. Unfortunately, this is a not true, because bacteria that cause serious infections are associated with mild fever.

Bacteria cannot survive if the temperature increases above 38°C, and will release toxins that block the brains temperature control area, the hypothalamus. Viruses can tolerate higher temperatures, and so boiling instruments does not kill viruses.

Please consult a doctor and actively look for the focus of infections that may require specific antibiotics.

Most doctors have a habit of giving broad-spectrum antibiotics because they have no clue about the specific bacteria causing an infection.

Evidence based medicine may say that 80% of patients with throat pain have streptococcus bacteria in the throat, so the treatment advised is penicillin. But if you are one of the 20% who had Mycoplasma, Haemophilus B, staphylococcus, or resistant pneumococcus instead, then the chances of you developing serious complications and dying is very high.

Wrong diagnoses and offering antibiotic prescriptions based only on evidence based medicine, resulting in colonization with antibiotic resistant bacteria, must be stopped. If the antibiotics, dose and method of administration are not correct, the bacteria will soon enter the blood stream, producing septicaemia (blood poisoning).

Please consult a doctor as soon as possible if you think you are unwell, and do not seek help from nurses, chemists, family or friends if you have symptoms that suggest an infection, because diagnosing infections is not simple, is riddled with questions we cannot answer, and has become a major threat to our profession.

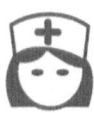 ## FEVER VERY HIGH

Parents get anxious because they associate a high fever with fits. Fits occur when the body temperature increases rapidly.

In the last thirty years of medical practice, we have never seen one child develop fits because the body temperature was very high.

Most mothers of children who were brought to hospital with fits felt guilty when we told them the fever was the cause of the fits.

The reason they could not identify this was because the body temperature rapidly increased, precipitating a fit. It is difficult to prevent fits associated with fever.

Please DO NOT distress a child by trying to check their temperature if you feel the body is very warm. This may raise the body temperature higher, and also precipitate a fit.

If you have identified fever in a child, please follow the instructions listed below and do not panic.

Please do not distress a febrile child just to record the temperature as it is not essential, but make sure you give them paracetamol or junifen for two to three days.

Please go to hospital, or call 999, because convulsions can occur again.

Do not switch on a fan or try giving a bath using TEPID SPONGING or LUKEWARM WATER. If you rapidly reduce the body temperature, the child may develop fits.

Please give anti-pyretic or non-steroid anti-inflammatory drugs regularly, as advised in the bottle or instructed by your doctor. The antipyretics can only suppress body temperature for 4–6 hours, and so the fever will bounce back when the drug wears off. The temperature will only return to normal and stay normal once the infection is cured.

Please note that an infection suppressed using low dose antibiotics will often return with a vengeance, and this time it will be because the bacteria have developed resistance. Please check the prescribed dosage, frequency, and duration of treatment, and follow these instructions meticulously.

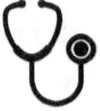 **FITS**

Also called convulsions. Fits is a common word used to explain fainting, epilepsy and convulsions.

Convulsions typically have three stages: acute rigidity, loss of consciousness, and a generalized tonic and clonic stage (stiffness and relaxation), resulting in a shaking episode and subsequent drifting to sleep.

Parents get anxious when their child develops high fever, because fits are associated with fever.

Fits occur when the body temperature increases rapidly (suddenly).

Most mothers of children who were brought to hospital with fits felt guilty when we told them the fever was the cause of the fits.

The reason they could not identify this was because the body temperature rapidly increased, precipitating a fit. It is difficult to prevent fits associated with fever.

If you have identified fever in a child, please follow the instructions in the notes and do not panic.

Please do not distress a febrile child just to record the temperature as it is not essential, but make sure you give them paracetamol or junifen for two to three days.

In the case of fit/convulsions, make sure that the patient is breathing, and feel the pulse rate. Do not try to put any object into the mouth. Fits will continue for a few minutes and they will then enter a relaxed state. Please go to hospital, or call 999, because convulsions can occur again.

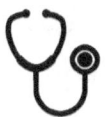 **FLUSH - FEELING OR LOOK FLUSHED**

A flushed look occurs because the circulation in the skin is increased.

You may also be sweaty and have palpitations.

If the core temperature (temperature in the body) is increased, chemicals are released by the brain to help increase circulation and open up sweat glands in the skin.

You will be sweaty, may feel hot or cold, and will have an increased pulse rate.

Please associate two other symptoms with this before rushing to a hospital or clinic, because you may be flushed because you are excited, sexually aroused, or even when you are just flirting.

This may be an exaggerated normal physiological response. This is likely to be caused by bacteria, viruses and allergies.

You must always speak to a doctor or call emergency nurse triage.

 **FLU**

The flu is the one of the most commonly occurring illness in the entire world, with more than 1 billion colds per year reported in the United States alone.

Flu is a self-limiting illness caused by any one of more than 200 viruses. The common cold produces mild symptoms usually lasting only 5–10 days. In contrast, the type of flu known as influenza, which is caused by a different class of virus, can have severe symptoms.

This must not be labeled as an illness disease to describe a combination of symptoms that has no treatment, e.g., a runny nose, fever, bodily pain, and coughing. To stop abusing antibiotics, the doctors must start making the correct diagnosis of rhinitis, tonsillitis, pharyngitis, sinusitis, pneumonias or atypical pneumonia, and prescribe the right antibiotics, not broad-spectrum antibiotics.

Some authors of medical textbooks have listed the "Common cold" as an infection caused by various viruses. In the past, this word was probably used to describe Asthma (Chronic Obstructive Lung Disease).

Please consult doctors to get the right diagnosis and treatment.

Do not abuse antibiotics. It is not good for you to take them unnecessarily, because your body will then become colonized with antibiotic resistant bacteria.

If you have recurrent coughs and colds, it is likely you are suffering because you are allergic to something, or are an undiagnosed asthmatic.

Please choose three symptoms that you have, and follow the instructions as described below.

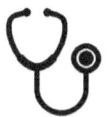 ## FOUL SMELLING VAGINAL DISCHARGE

Chronic foul smelling vaginal discharge is called pelvic inflammatory disease (PID), and is an infection of the womb (uterus and/or fallopian tubes).

Pain in the lower abdomen (pelvic area) is the most common symptom. It can range from mild to severe.

Pain and/or bleeding during sex can also occur.

Chlamydia, gonococcus, syphilis, staphylococcus, E. Coli and other bacteria can thrive in the womb, and will be difficult to treat. You must consult a gynaecologist or a sexually transmitted disease specialist in the genitourinary department (GUM Clinic) to identify the organisms involved, and determine the antibiotic that is required.

This infection can be treated using the right antibiotics. If it is not, women can develop infertility, or have serious problems during pregnancy.

We anticipate that this will be a major problem in the future, because treatment resistant gonococcus, chlamydia, and syphilis are coming back with a vengeance.

Teenagers have become more sexually active in the last ten years. As a result, incidences of these infections have rapidly increased in the western world.

Please consult a gynaecologist, or go to a GUM clinic, because the long-term problems like infertility and other problems associated with PID will be difficult to manage.

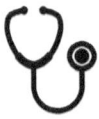

FRESH BLOOD IN STOOL

Fresh blood in stool, fresh blood dripping from the anus is often not very serious, because blood drips from cuts and fissures that are present in and around the anus. Internal bleeding usually produces a stool. Colonoscopy or sigmoidoscopy and blood tests are often not necessary.

Please do not panic and rush to a hospital. Speak to your doctors, or consult a nurse. All that you will need is someone to look at your anus, and maybe perform an internal examination. This will be embarrassing, but necessary. There are creams and suppositories that can usually resolve this common symptom.

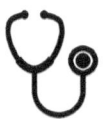

GASTRIC ULCER

This may be caused by an infection, so please do not self-diagnose yourself based on this symptom.

With a gastric ulcer, constant pain or cramps can occur, which are particularly bad after eating (eating tends to settle pain in a duodenal ulcer).

Indigestion remedies (antacids) often settle the pain, but it invariably returns. Belching is common and embarrassing.

Vomiting can occur.

Most people know they have developed a duodenal ulcer at around 2 am when they wake with a pain like a red-hot poker just above the belly button. Drinking milk can help, but hot spicy foods make it much worse. Eating small amounts of food often relieves the pain.

Ulcers may be caused by a bacterium called helicobacter that lives in the stomach. Your doctor can check for this. Stress, smoking, and alcohol abuse may also be contributing causes.

To prevent ulcers, you should avoid smoking and excessive indulgence in alcohol and 'rich' foods. Milk and indigestion remedies (antacids) do help. Possible complications are blood, or brown soil-like bloody vomit, the presence of black, tar-like blood or fresh red blood in your stools, and severe pain just below the rib cage.

You may feel dizziness when standing up, and a strong urge to drink, because you are thirsty.

Most peptic ulcers will respond well to treatment with modern drugs which reduce the amount of stomach acid.

You can also help ease the pain by using indigestion remedies or antacids.

If the incidents of pain have not just started, but have lasted more than a week, despite medicines from your pharmacist, call your doctor.

If the pain does not get better after 15–20 minutes, think of a heart attack, call 999, and go to hospital.

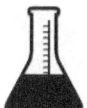

GASTRITIS

Gastritis is more common in middle aged people, after heavy meals or alcohol consumption, and is often worse at night. Regurgitation or reflux is painful, although rarely dangerous.

Stomach acid escapes into the gullet, causing chest pain. It can be mistaken for a heart attack, or vice versa.

This is a vague pain below the ribcage, extending into the throat, accompanied by an acid taste in the mouth, and excessive wind.

This classically occurs after a heavy meal or drinking alcohol, consuming rich food, often with a high fat content, excessive smoking, or as a result of a leaking valve at the neck of the stomach (hiatus hernia).

Prevent this by avoiding food which you know provokes an attack, sleeping with your upper body propped up with pillows, avoiding eating just before bed time, and eating small meals more often.

Avoid aspirin and drugs like nurofen, diclofenac, and ibuprofen (Non-Steroidal Anti-inflammatory drugs).

Most indigestion is harmless but annoying.

The acid refluxing into the throat does not appear to cause any serious damage. The greatest danger is ignoring repeated attacks, confusing them with a heart attack, or assuming gastritis and missing the signs of a heart attack.

Go to A&E if your symptoms persist or get worse after 15–20 minutes. Please do not think the doctors will get annoyed if you present yourself with chest pain and it turns out to be gastritis, but they will not be pleased if you go to A&E when the complications of a heart attack have already set in.

Your pharmacist will advise you about indigestion remedies (antacids and other medicines). Please take Gaviscon advance, and not powders or tablets.

Avoid taking large amounts of sodium bicarbonate (bicarbonate of soda), as this is turned into salt in the body.

If this is an on-going problem, please consult a doctor to get tested to rule out a helicobacter infection.

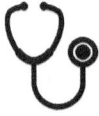 ## GENITAL BLISTERS

One in six Americans were found to be infected with genital herpes. About sixteen percent of Americans between the ages of 14 and 49 are affected, making it one of the most common sexually transmitted diseases in the USA.

About twenty-one percent (21%) of women were infected with genital herpes, compared to only eleven percent (11.5%) of men. Eight out of ten people with genital herpes do not know they are infected.

There is no cure for genital herpes or the herpes simplex virus type 2 (HSV-2), which can cause recurrent and painful genital sores, and increases the likelihood of acquiring and transmitting the AIDS virus.

It is related to herpes simplex virus 1, or oral herpes, which causes cold sores.

Because herpes is so prevalent, you must use condoms consistently and correctly with all of your sexual partners.

The CDC estimates that there are 19 million new infections of sexually transmitted disease every year in the United States, costing the health care system about $16 billion annually.

This symptom refers to intensely painful ulcers or blisters on the genitalia that may be recurrent. These are commonly a result of unprotected sex.

There are very few treatment options, and you should go to a genitourinary clinic (GU) or sexually transmitted disease (STD) walk-in-clinic.

 **GERMAN MEASLES (Rubella)**

This disease was uncommon, thanks to the Measles, Mumps and Rubella (MMR) vaccine but seems likely to return with a vengeance.

The person is rarely ill, but will have a slightly raised temperature and swollen glands on the neck and base of the skull.

The pinhead sized flat, red spots last around two days and need no treatment. Paracetamol will help reduce the slight fever.

This virus is very contagious, and will spread quickly in a population which is not immune.

Vaccination for girls and boys is both safe and effective.

Complications are very rare, but can include encephalitis (inflammation of the brain)

The real danger may come in later life. If an unvaccinated woman becomes infected with German Measles (Rubella) while pregnant, it can affect the development of the baby. For this major reason alone, both boys and girls should be immunized with this very safe vaccine.

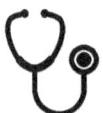

GREEN COLORED (BILE VOMIT)

The most common causes of this symptom are an infection or an obstruction in the intestine.

The problem is how to differentiate between bacterial and viral infections, obstructions, and metabolic, liver, or gall bladder problems.

The diagnosis of this symptom requires proper clinical examination, will require investigation, and probably admission to hospital.

Doctors will only treat this symptom after ruling out serious illnesses, so please consult a DOCTOR and not a nurse in the UK.

Please do not panic, but go to A&E if you cannot get an appointment, or you cannot speak to or consult a doctor.

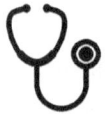

HANGOVER

A hangover can be so bad you think there is something seriously wrong with you, especially if it is the first time it has ever happened to you.

A headache, nausea, tiredness, and thirst are the commonest symptoms. Dehydration is the main cause. Alcohol acts as a diuretic, stimulating the kidneys to lose water.

Some alcoholic drinks contain toxins, which act as mild poisons. Red wine in excess tends to cause headaches for this reason.

Sleep while intoxicated is always poor, as the alcohol interferes with the normal sleep pattern. This causes a feeling of not having slept the next morning. Vomiting when asleep can result in aspiration and death, because the reflexes are inhibited, and you may die due to anoxia (loss of oxygen supply).

Obviously, the best way to avoid a hangover is not to drink to excess. Drinking a few glasses of water before retiring will also help. Switch to less strong or non-alcoholic drinks towards the end of the evening.

Hangovers are rarely dangerous, but routinely taking "a hair of the dog" to ease the symptoms can lead to alcohol abuse. People underestimate just how long alcohol stays in the blood stream after a night's drinking, and may well be still over the legal limit for driving the next day.

Drink plenty of water, take some paracetamol, and if possible have a nap later on to make up for the poor quality of your sleep. You can also drink Coca Cola or Pepsi Cola with two, three or four pinches of salt per can or glass. The cola must be flat, and this will quickly rehydrate you and help to reduce the headache.

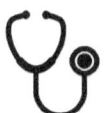

HEAD ACHE

A headache is considered a common modern day illness, and too many people waste time and money trying to identify the cause, requesting investigations and abusing drugs.

An acute headache associated with a viral illness or sinusitis is by far the commonest cause of a headache, but some doctors and patients assume tension and migraine headaches as the commonest cause in general practice.

We do not label headaches as a common symptom that can be managed with self-medication, because missing a sign of illnesses like high blood pressure, temporal arteritis, and some other rare conditions can result in long-term complications, blindness, and even death.

Every patient complaining of a headache must first get their blood pressure checked by a doctor (3 times on alternate weeks).

Irritability increases with a headache, along with a greater risk of having an accident, and the risk of overdosing on paracetamol.

If the cause is obvious, doctors will reassure the patient and explain it, or will suggest simple analgesics, e.g., taking ibuprofen if you have only tried paracetamol so far. An over-enthusiastic urge to investigate can often result in stress (waiting for test results, being told the blood test is not conclusive, or having doctors label you as mildly hypertensive, etc.), making the symptom get worse.

You must treat the following headaches as Emergency and go to hospital:

If there is a mild fever, rash (that does not fade with pressure) and vomiting, you must always think of meningitis. These patients will have neck stiffness – being unable to bend it to touch their chin on their chest, or not being able to bend and kiss their knee. Babies will not turn their heads to look at you, and are often very irritable with a high pitched cry.

A sudden or sub-acute "thunderclap" or squeezing type headache can be accompanied by neurological symptoms, such as weakness on one side, blindness, and loss of sensation.

The regular use of analgesics with codeine may cause analgesic headaches.

If you are over 50 years old and have unexplained headaches, it is possible to suspect temporal arteritis or acute glaucoma (if you have a visual acuity problem, this can result in blindness if it is not managed well)

Carbon monoxide poisoning presents with a headache.

A subarachnoid hemorrhage shows as a sudden, severe pain situated in the base of skull behind the neck.

If this symptom does not resolve after taking painkillers like analgesics, you must consult a doctor to get a proper clinical examination, check your blood pressure, and check your eyes with a funduscopy.

Please do not panic, but go to A&E if you cannot get an appointment or you cannot speak to or consult a doctor.

The majority of people with a headache think it is a migraine, and often waste time and consult the doctor late. It is important to check your blood pressure if you have a recurrent headache.

Stroke and internal bleeding can be reduced if you consult a doctor or a nurse to get a BP check.

Please consult a nurse if this is the only symptom. If there are other associated symptoms, you may have a serious problem, so please consult a doctor or go to A&E.

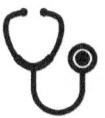 **HEAD INJURY**

The seriousness of this symptom depends on the circumstances. How did it happen? Was there any loss of consciousness, confusion, convulsions, amnesia or vomiting?

This can be associated with headaches, drowsiness, neurological disturbance (e.g., numbness, paralysis, double vision), bleeding disorder, anticoagulants, and recent alcohol or recreational drug use.

Is the patient still confused or drowsy?

Look at the injury and see if there is a dent or swelling.

Check pupils: Shine a light in the patient's eyes, and see if their pupils are equal, and whether they react to light.

Is it painful to the patient when you shine bright lights on their eyes (photophobia)?

Go to hospital if the injury was a high-energy impact to head, and the patient lost consciousness or has amnesia; if you are confused, or had convulsions (fits); if there is reason to suspect a skull fracture (orbital herniation, deafness, clear cerebrospinal fluid secreted from the ear or nose); if there are signs of substance intoxication, neurological disturbance, or unequal pupils; if the patient has a bleeding disorder, or is on anticoagulants; or if there is no one to supervise the patient at home.

An injury or blow to the head will cause a concussion. The seriousness of the concussion depends upon the severity of the injury. Nearly all patients with even slight concussion will have a headache for 48 hours. Some may well feel a little washed out and irritable during this period.

Children often feel sick, and may vomit and appear to be sleepy. This is to be expected in children who have had a blow to the head, and lasts for 12–24 hours.

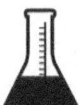 ## HEAD LICE

These tiny parasites can live on any hairy part of the body. Female lice lay eggs every day. The eggs hatch in 8–10 days.

Lice are nearly always completely harmless, but terribly itchy. Lice and their eggs (nits) can be seen on the hair shafts.

Social status means nothing to lice. They are very common among children, and an infestation has nothing to do with dirty living.

Lice are easily caught from others. Avoid spreading lice by treating the whole family at once. Avoid lending or borrowing hats, brushes or combs, and keep hair clean.

As lice can stay alive for two days when they are not on a human being, thoroughly clean clothes and hats which have been worn, as well as combs and brushes.

To prevent lice, comb the hair regularly while wet with a fine-toothed comb. Use a conditioner to make combing easier.

The safest and most effective treatment is daily combing with a nit comb. Use only conditioner and a nit comb, or ask your pharmacist for further advice.

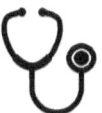 HEART BURN

The most common cause of this is gastritis.

Heartburn is sudden onset, sharp, excruciating pain in the chest, commonly on the left side of the chest, just below the nipple, a burning sensation behind the breast bone which is made worse by stooping or lying flat.

There may also be an acid taste brought up from the stomach.

You may have difficulty in swallowing with repeated reflux of stomach acid.

Heartburn that does not resolve within 15 minutes after taking an antacid is an emergency. You must CALL 999 and go to the nearest hospital A&E. Please do not expect that a visiting doctor can manage this symptom at home – this will cause you to waste your valuable minutes.

Please do not drive. Call an ambulance if the associated symptoms are red, and treat this as an emergency.

Heartburn is caused due to reflux – the bringing up of stomach acid into the gullet. This condition used to be more than just a nuisance before the appearance of modern drugs, which reduce the production of stomach acid.

A hiatus hernia causes the neck of the stomach to roll into the chest, allowing stomach acid to pass into the gullet.

You can't prevent a hiatus hernia but you can ease the symptoms. You can prevent many of the symptoms by controlling your weight, controlling how much you eat, and not smoking. Avoid foods that trigger off attacks – such as rich and fatty foods. Take indigestion remedies (antacids), and drink milk to relieve the symptoms. Sleep with an extra pillow to stop the acid reflux.

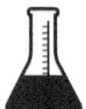 **HEAT RASH**

All babies and children will at some time have a rash that we call heat rash. It looks like a fine pattern of tiny red spots, which come and go, but tend to disappear if their temperature is lowered. The baby will otherwise be perfectly well.

A cold (viral infection) is the most common cause.

Too many clothes or bedding will also cause this rash to appear. If babies get too hot, cool them down immediately by removing their clothes and keeping them in a cool room.

No treatment is required other than lowering their temperature with Paracetamol syrup (e.g. Calpol).

High fever (over 38°C or 100.4°F) is often seen in viral infections because viruses are not killed by very high temperature.

Please note that high fever can change in hours, so please use MAYA and check again using the changed symptom.

Please do not make the child cry and get anxious because you want to check their temperature. If the child is crying the body temperature and heart rate (pulse) will increase, and this can precipitate fits.

When you give Paracetamol, please GIVE THIS REGULARLY, 4–6 hourly or as instructed on the bottle. Do not get anxious about giving too much paracetamol for 2–3 days, as, if you give too little, the consequences and probable hospitalization are more dangerous than the drug. The drugs have been used for long time and are safe. This drug works for only 4–6 hours. You must also check the dosage – if you give less than is advised, the drugs will not work.

You can also try Non-Steroidal Anti-Inflammatory drugs (Brufen, Junifen) twice daily to help reduce a temperature. Giving a lukewarm water bath is safer, and probably better than drugs. The body is trying to reduce its core temperature, and lukewarm water opens the sweat glands and reduces body temperature.

Please do not give aspirin to children.

Give the child plenty of drinks (water, juice or even flat coke). If the child refuses to eat solids, please do not get worried and force feed the child. As long as the child or you drink fluids, you will not be deprived of food and be hungry. (Please Read "Dehydration")

We have seen children with severe dehydration admitted into hospital because the parents were not giving them fluids to drink but forcing them to eat solids. So PLEASE GIVE FLUIDS – FLUIDS, FLUIDS, and MORE FLUIDS.

Do not use aromatic oils to help with breathing, or give cough mixtures to suppress a cough. Babies do not know how to breathe through their mouth and so will find it hard to breathe at all.

If you are worried or the symptoms are getting worse please speak to your doctors first, and do not rush to hospital.

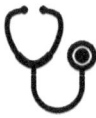 HIGH PITCHED CRY

This is one symptom I always worry about because of two reasons, (1) the mother is distressed and no one can make her relaxed, and (2) it is difficult to examine this child and find out what is the cause.

The most common causes in babies are a blocked nose causing anoxia and a headache, an intestinal obstruction or colic (due to a rumbling intestine that may be scary, though intestinal hurry is not said to be painful).

If you have ruled out hunger, thirst, a wet nappy, constipation, or a urinary infection, then we need to examine and investigate the baby after he or she settles down.

Give paracetamol or Calpol to see if the child settles. If he or she stops crying, the cause of the cry is pain, but we need to identify the cause of the pain. You must always consult a doctor to find the cause of this pain. Please read the information on abdominal pain, because we do not think it is a good idea to suppress a symptom without knowing the origin of the pain. Pain may come back and also lead to complications.

Babies often develop a headache if they have difficulty breathing, croup, or blocked nostrils. In future we need to also be aware of epiglottitis.

Some children with syndromes may have an irritable cry, but the parents will know about this.

People assume pulling the leg up and crying is associated with the baby having tummy pain. This is not 100% true, but some babies with urine infections and/or constipation do have tummy pain.

Common causes like an ear infection, nappy rash, hunger, urinary tract infections, and thrush are easy to diagnose.

Doctors do not know what causes colic. But we have noticed that babies with poor feeding technique cry. The most common cause of excessive crying is air phage, i.e., sucking in air when feeding. This happens when the teat of the bottle has a small hole. Babies get tired, open their mouth in between feeds, and swallow air. Trapped wind will stretch the stomach and produce a rumbling noise that may be painful. This can also happen when the mouth is not properly latched onto the nipple of the breast.

Please check the associated symptoms before rushing to hospital.

Please note that some babies (more boys than girls) develop projectile vomiting because they have developed a tightening of the stomach (pyloric stenosis), and are often very hungry, but they do not have a high pitched cry because the stenosis is not painful.

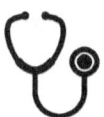

HOARSE VOICE

This is associated with pharyngitis, or a problem in the vocal cords.

If you have a fever, then the most likely cause is pharyngitis.

You need specific antibiotics and may require investigation and referral to a specialist.

An abscess in the throat known as quincy can also alter the voice. This problem may require hospital treatment.

The diagnosis of this symptom requires proper clinical examination, and may require investigation.

Doctors will only treat this symptom after ruling out serious illnesses, so you must consult a DOCTOR.

Please do not panic, but go to A&E or the ER if you cannot get an appointment or you cannot speak to or consult a doctor.

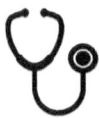 ## HOT AND SWEATY

The cause of this symptom may be an infection or hyper dynamic circulation.

This is likely to be a chronic problem and not necessarily an acute one that must be treated as an emergency.

The key is to differentiate between endocrinal causes, deficiencies, and bacterial or viral infections.

The diagnosis of this symptom requires proper clinical examination, and may require investigation.

Doctors will only treat this symptom after ruling out serious illnesses so please consult a DOCTOR.

Please do not panic, but go to A&E or the ER if you cannot get an appointment or you cannot speak to or consult a doctor.

 ## IMPETIGO

Bacterial infections of the skin are fairly common. Impetigo is more common in children, but is also seen in adults.

It is infectious, but is no longer a serious threat, thanks to antibiotics.

It usually begins as a small red spot, which gradually increases in size.

The top then becomes crusty and weeps.

It is often found around the corners of the mouth, and on the face, but can also be found on the rest of the body.

It is infectious, and is caught from direct contact with infected children or adults. It is also spread through the sharing of face cloths and towels.

It spreads much more quickly between people who are generally run down as a result of illness or stress.

Clean the spots with a damp tissue. Give painkillers like Paracetamol for any pain. Antibiotic creams will be needed.

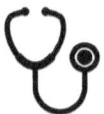

IMPOTENCY

Erectile dysfunction (ED), or impotence, is a sexual dysfunction characterized by the inability to develop or maintain an erection of the penis during sexual intercourse.

A penile erection occurs when the blood enters the cavernous (sponge-like bodies) tissue within the penis. This process is initiated as a result of sexual arousal, when signals are transmitted from the brain via the nerves.

Diseases or disorders of the cardiovascular, or metabolic systems, and hormonal or neurological abnormalities can produce ED.

Drugs and psychological problems are more important than physiological problems in this case. ED can result in relationship difficulties and damage to the masculine self-image.

Besides treating the underlying causes such as potassium deficiency, or arsenic contamination of drinking water, the first-line treatments of erectile dysfunction consist of a trial of drugs like sildenafil (Viagra), which helps establish the cause.

Approximately 40% of males suffer from erectile dysfunction or impotence, at least occasionally.

Please consult your doctors and get help.

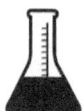 **INDIGESTION**

Indigestion is a term people can use to refer to tummy pain, gastritis, and even diarrhoea and vomiting. It is essential that you specify the symptom and not simply say "indigestion" because this is not a disease or a symptom that a doctor can clearly define.

Acid reflux is more common in middle aged people, occurs most frequently after heavy meals or alcohol consumption and is often worse at night. This regurgitation or reflux of acid can be painful, although rarely dangerous. It is more properly called esophagitis, or "heartburn" (see above). Stomach acid escapes into the gullet causing chest pain. It can be mistaken for a heart attack.

Severe reflux can occur with a hiatus hernia, vague pain below the ribcage, extending into the throat, an acid taste in the mouth, and passing excessive wind (please read about "Irritable Bowel Syndrome").

This form of indigestion classically occurs after a heavy meal or drinking alcohol, eating 'rich' food, often with a high fat content, and/or excessive smoking.

Avoid aspirin and drugs like ibuprofen (Non-Steroidal Anti-inflammatory drugs).

Most indigestion is harmless, but annoying. The acid refluxing into the throat does not appear to cause any serious damage. The greatest danger is ignoring repeated attacks, or confusing it with a heart attack. Obtain medical advice if your symptoms persist or get worse.

Your pharmacist will give you advice about indigestion remedies (antacids and other medicines).

Avoid taking large amounts of sodium bicarbonate (bicarbonate of soda), as this is turned into salt in the body.

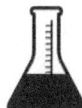 **INJURY MINOR**

Management of injuries depends on the severity of the injury, the impairment of function, and the age and relevant medical history of the patient.

Minor injury in healthy young adults can be managed at home using an ice pack (e.g., pack of frozen peas, wrapped in a towel,) to help reduce swelling and pain.

Try topical NSAID (Non-steroidal Anti-Inflammatory Drugs) for soft tissue injuries (e.g., ibuprofen or voltarol emugel) if the injury is small.

Ibuprofen or voltarol can be taken orally after food if you do not suffer from gastritis, recurrent tummy pain, or have any history of ulcers.

Mobilize injured arms, legs or joints only after 48 hours rest, or when the pain has reduced after taking anti-inflammatory drugs.

Compression may be a valuable early treatment for joint injuries, with the exception of the ankle, where there is no evidence that it will benefit from elevation above the level of the heart.

You must consult a doctor in hospital if you have developed a deformity, have severe pain, bony tenderness, are unable to bear weight on a leg, or have severe bleeding.

Minor bleeding can be stopped using a tourniquet or pressure bandage.

Please do go to A&E and do not wait for an appointment at your GP surgery or a home visit if you think there may be a fracture or the injury is serious.

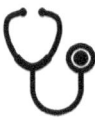 **INJURY SEVERE**

Management of an injury depends on the severity of bleeding, in the injury.

Go to A&E if you have been involved in a road traffic accident, have serious bleeding, if your injury is associated with an impairment of function, or impacts another existing medical condition.

If you are on drugs like anticoagulants or immune-suppressants, receiving cancer treatment, or develop swelling rapidly or gradually, you must consult a doctor or go to hospital.

If the injury is gradually developing swelling, deformity, bony tenderness, and restriction of movement, go to A&E.

If the bleeding is severe, please DO NOT take Ibuprofen or Voltarol, because these drugs can produce gastric irritation resulting in bleeding.

All serious injuries and severe bleeding require you to call an ambulance and consult a doctor in hospital.

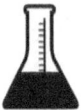 **INSECT BITE**

An insect bite (mosquito, ant, bee, wasp or others) produces a local reaction like pain, swelling and itching.

This usually resolves after you take an antihistamine or antibiotic cream.

Insect bites are not to be dismissed as minor. The bacteria, viruses and fungi transferred by insects are becoming lethal killers because they are resistant to treatment, and so they can be very important.

Please note that symptoms can change any time from day one to a few days after the bite. If you develop a generalized reaction a few days later, please speak to doctors.

You may have been bitten by mosquitoes a few weeks ago but then developed other symptoms like feeling hot and cold. This might be malaria. You must consult doctors and get a blood test to help get a clear diagnosis.

The generalized reaction is more serious, and must be managed in hospital as an emergency.

Please choose symptoms that are associated with this one. If you do not have any associated symptoms, then the problem is unlikely to be serious. You can consult a chemist who can give you the required treatment.

If two associated symptoms are RED, PLEASE TREAT THIS AS AN EMERGENCY AND GO TO HOSPITAL. PLEASE DO NOT DRIVE, CALL AN AMBULANCE.

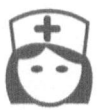 ## INSOMNIA

Food, water, oxygen, and sleep are essential for humans and animals to live.

A lack of sleep makes you lethargic, unable to concentrate, have mood swings, and also develop other illnesses due to hormonal imbalance.

Some people require only four or five hours' sleep a night, whereas others need ten hours or more.

The amount of sleep required tends to lessen with age, and also with lower activity levels. A 'good night's sleep' is not the same for everyone. People who are burnt out often have sleep problems.

Almost everyone will have periods of insomnia at some stage. Extroverts are alert during the night and so work more at night. They often sleep once every two or three days for 12–18 hours. This is called catch-up sleep and rarely needs treatment.

REM (Rapid Eye Movement) sleep is important. This is the last stage of sleep. People who do not get REM often find it hard to relax, and may lack energy and feel they are depressed.

Early morning waking is a good indication that you may be depressed.

You need to answer the following questions:

What is your concern about the sleeping pattern?

When did this problem start, and what else was happening at that time?

Are you finding it difficult getting off to sleep?

Are you waking up often during the night?

Are you waking up in the early morning feeling tired?

What was your previous pattern like?

Do you take daytime naps?

Does your partner say that you snore and are restless?

What are your expectations of treatment?

Common causes are: Excessive caffeine, nicotine, alcohol, recreational drugs, and lifestyle factors – e.g., shift work.

A more complete list of potential causes is given below:

Physical: pain, itching, shortness of breath, nocturia, indigestion, tinnitus, discomfort, too warm, too cold, noise, room not dark enough.

Physiological: shift work, jet lag, and pregnancy.

Psychological: emotional upsets, worries, and bereavement.

Psychiatric: especially depression, or hypomania.

Pathological: sleep apnoea, restless leg syndrome.

Pharmacological: is the patient on any medication which might cause insomnia, e.g., corticosteroids, propranolol, pseudoephedrine or laxatives, or taking in excessive levels of coffee, tea, cola, alcohol, or nicotine?

Social: presence of a new baby, shift work, enuretic child, partner who has nocturia or who snores.

Are you agitated, depressed or anxious and feel 'washed out'?

If you are obese this can be associated with sleep apnoea syndrome.

Deal with the underlying cause, where possible.

Avoid going to bed until you feel sleepy.

Take a warm, milky drink before bedtime.

Regular exercise is helpful, but not just before bedtime.

Relaxation exercises or training (e.g., hypnotherapy) can be helpful; also yoga, meditation, reading, and listening to relaxing music.

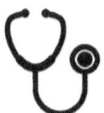 **IRRITABILITY**

Irritability is a useful sign in children.

Babies who are anoxic (lack oxygen supply to brain), hungry, or develop pain in their tummy or head are often irritable.

Excessive crying, a high pitched cry, and not settling are a good indication that something is not right.

We have noticed that babies of a mother who is stressed or postnatally depressed, or who is having family problems are often irritable.

Babies of mothers who are trying to breast feed and getting stressed will also become irritable. This may be because they are not getting enough breast milk, or their sucking technique is bad and they swallow air and develop colic and low blood sugar.

Teenagers and children with learning difficulties can get frustrated, have low self-esteem, and therefore become irritable, have temper tantrums, and often get into fights with their peers.

Adults who are stressed because of work, family problems and financial difficulties, are manic or depressed, are frustrated and so have mood swings, a lack of sleep, and poor concentration. They are snappy or mute, but get very irritated with minor problems.

We have marked this red, as it is an important sign, and you must consult a doctor soon.

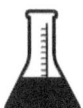 IRRITABLE BOWEL

The cause of this remains unknown though it is a common complaint.

Diagnosis is based on patient history, and the exclusion of any other potential conditions.

There is no definitive test for irritable bowel syndrome (IBS). It affects three times as many women as men.

Symptoms can start at any age but predominantly appear in persons between 15 and 40 years old. Stress and lifestyle are major factors.

Common Presentation: If you are passing excessive wind (flatus), have intermittent constipation or diarrhoea, a colicky tummy (on and off abdominal pain), and feel your tummy is bloated, you are likely to have IBS.

The cause of this illness is unknown, but it may be stress related or because your tummy is colonized with bad bacteria (common after taking antibiotics).

You can prevent this by having a high-fibre diet containing wholegrain bread, rice, and pasta. Eating plenty of fresh fruit can produce a remarkable long-term improvement in symptoms. Dairy products are often the worst.

Try eliminating cheese, milk, chocolate, butter and cream from your diet for a few weeks to see if there is any improvement.

All red meat, not just beef, can often seriously upset your bowel if you are prone to IBS.

Use herbs known to alleviate the symptoms of IBS, e.g., peppermint. Stress can be a big factor.

Exercise increases bowel activity, thus reducing bloating and distension. Nicotine stimulates receptors in the bowel which can make your IBS much worse.

Small amounts of alcohol can actually help to stimulate gentle bowel function.

Tea contains as much caffeine as coffee. Both, therefore, stimulate bowel action resulting in diarrhoea in the susceptible person. Coffee also contains an unknown substance that causes bowel cramps.

Drugs are the last resort, and will only have a temporary effect. Codeine relieves the spasm, but can cause constipation. Peppermint oil is the base ingredient of many drugs prescribed for IBS.

Buscopan often helps to reduce spasmodic pain, but ibuprofen can produce gastritis and so you should avoid this drug. Paracetamol rarely helps ease pain.

Anti-diarrhoeal drugs and laxatives can help, but long-term use of these is not good.

The pain and discomfort of IBS can sometimes be relieved by a hot water bottle, which fits nice and snugly against your stomach.

However, see your doctor if: the home treatment doesn't work, after two weeks you pass blood in your motions, your bowel motions are very dark black or covered with mucus, or there is an unexplained weight loss.

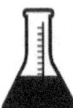

ITCHING AFTER HOT BATH

This rash is reddish, and very itchy in the night.

It is not an emergency, but requires the right treatment, otherwise the infestation will spread in your family and community.

If the doctor or nurse has diagnosed this symptom as eczema, and you are on steroid cream, please stop using this and consult a dermatologist.

This is a typical case of a rash appearing on your skin when you sleep in bed. The cause is usually bed bugs and scabies.

You must clear the bacterial infection first, and then start antifungal treatment.

Please make sure every person living in your house is treated with the drug on the same day.

Wash all your clothes and bed linen in a hot wash on the day you take the treatment.

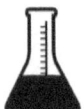

ITCHY ANUS

This is called as pruritus ani. It is common in children infested with worms like pinworm.

Please check the bottom to see if there are burrows or a rash.

The worms lay eggs around the anus, and often enter the vagina. This can spread from hand to mouth.

Please ask a chemist to advise treatment.

Please treat other children and adults living in the same house.

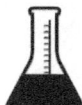 ## ITCHY LUMPS ON LEGS AND ARMS

At first, insect bites can be mistaken for more serious things.

If you look very closely you can generally see the small hole of the actual bite.

The rash or individual 'spot' is invariably itchy and may swell, particularly if it is a bite from a horse fly.

Causes: Midges, horse flies, bees, wasps, centipedes, ants, lice, etc. The list is long, and please check if there are any killer insects in the area you are living in. Local chemists may have this information, or you can find information on the Internet.

Public health officials have published a list of insects that may bite, and also provide information about treatment.

Prevention: Insect repellents work. If you suspect lice, ask your pharmacist for advice.

If you are swamped with bees or wasps, try switching off your mobile phone. The radio-magnetic waves emitted by the mobile phone can block magnetic waves that bees and wasp follow to go back home. They are then lost and so fly around your head trying to find their way.

Some people are strongly allergic to bites and stings and can become very ill. If there is any shortness of breath, dial 999. Scratching can infect bites.

Although itchy and sometimes painful they are rarely dangerous, and need only some antihistamine or local anaesthetic cream from your pharmacist.

The redness and swelling are usually due to the allergic reaction rather than to an infection. Antibiotics are rarely needed for swelling seen in the first 48 hours.

Call your doctor if the symptoms persist, or you have other associated symptoms that are RED.

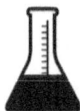 **ITCHY PENIS**

The most common cause of this is candida, a fungus which is normally present in large numbers in the vagina. For various reason it can grow rapidly and cause thrush in women and also infect men after sex.

Your partner may have a creamy discharge, itchiness and irritation in the vagina and pain or burning after passing water.

Check with your doctor if you are on steroid treatment or have diabetes.

Sexual intercourse with infected women is the most common cause of this.

Prevention: After being on the toilet, wipe from front to back. Change underwear frequently, particularly after exercise. Choose cotton rather than nylon pants. Avoid harsh soaps; they kill the good bacteria, which prevent thrush.

Complications: There are few serious complications of thrush but it can, however, make life very miserable. Sex is painful, as is passing water. This fungus has become resistant to treatment, so if the drugs have not helped, please consult a doctor.

Ask your pharmacist for antifungal preparations like miconazol or canistin.

Your partner may need treatment as well.

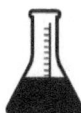 ## ITCHY RASH

Allergic reaction: This is probably the most common cause of itchy skin, and might also be accompanied by puffiness and redness around the eyes and lips.

Along with the itchiness there will also most probably be problems with breathing, throat and nose, and possibly even the head as well.

If the itchy rash is experienced mostly in the spring, the time that allergies often affect sufferers, or if you know that you have been exposed to something that you are allergic to, then it is pretty obvious what is causing the itching.

This rash blanches (fades) on pressure and can often be frightening to see.

The treatment is antihistamines. These can be bought in the chemist.

If breathlessness and swollen lips occur, you must rush to a hospital A&E.

Please consult a doctor soon to get tests and identify what you are allergic to. Some will not perform the tests, and simply making a note of substances you are allergic to is more than enough.

Eczema, Scabies, Fungus infections and liver disease also produce generalized itchy rash.

If itching is a problem during pregnancy, or after starting a new treatment, please consult your doctor. You will need a blood test and investigation to rule out serious illnesses that are associated with itching.

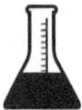 ITCHY VAGINA

Candida albicans is a fungus, which should not normally be present in large numbers in the vagina. For various reasons, it can grow rapidly and cause thrush.

Symptoms: A creamy thick white vaginal discharge. Itchiness and irritation, and pain or burning after passing water.

Common Causes:

- A prolonged course of antibiotics.
- The oral contraceptive pill.
- Hormonal changes preceding the period.
- Steroid treatment.
- Diabetes.
- Immune system problems.
- Sexual intercourse with an infected man.

Prevention: After being on the toilet, wipe from front to back. Change underwear frequently, particularly after exercise. Choose cotton rather than nylon pants. Avoid harsh soaps; they kill the good bacteria, which prevent thrush.

Complications: There are few serious complications of thrush but it can, however, make life very miserable. Sex is painful, as is passing water. This fungus has become resistant to treatment, so if the drugs have not helped, please consult a doctor.

Eat live yoghurt and apply it to the vaginal area. It will replace the missing Lactobacillus, which prevents thrush.

Ask your pharmacist for antifungal preparations like miconazol or canistin.

Your partner may need treatment as well.

If the discharge changes in smell or appearance, there is any abdominal pain, or the thrush either does not disappear after self-care or keeps coming back for no apparent reason, please consult your doctor.

PS: Candida is said to be resistant to treatment, so you may need different drugs and maybe oral antifungal drugs.

ITCHY AFTER HOT BATH

Although intensely itchy, mainly at night and after hot bath, this is not a serious problem. Common causes are scabies, bed bugs, and other infestations which kindle an allergic response and release histamines.

Scabies is caused by a mite, which burrows just under the skin, often between the fingers, on wrists, elbows and the genital areas causing a red rash. It can only come from contact with infected people. Red lines, which follow the burrows of the mite as it travels into the skin, soon merge with the inevitable scratching. It is usually worse at night when the mite is most active.

Bacterial infections from excessive scratching can make the situation worse.

Please do not use steroid cream, because this will help spread scabies, and a bacterial infection will occur.

Ointments are available from your pharmacist. All of the body will need to be covered with the ointment for 24 hours, and all clothing and bedding should be washed thoroughly.

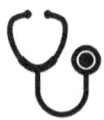

JAUNDICE

Having a yellow tinge to the whites of the eyes is often a sign that you have a mild attack of jaundice. If your eyes are yellow then it is quite likely that your skin will be too.

Jaundice is quite common in new-borns, but it can affect people at any age, and be variable in its intensity. If an affected baby is not feeding well, and is drowsy and lethargic, please consult a doctor because the baby may develop long-term problems. Please make sure the baby is feeding well, because low sugar will allow jaundice to enter the brain resulting in kernicterus.

Jaundice is what happens when bilirubin builds up in our body tissue and in the blood.

The most common causes for this build-up of bilirubin are a liver condition, such as hepatitis, or the presence of gallstones.

If you have a yellowing of the whites of the eyes as well as a tinge of yellow to your skin, also look at the mucous membranes of the nose and mouth, which may also have taken on a yellow hue. This is cirrhosis of the liver.

When you go to the toilet, you might notice that the urine you pass is darker in color, and that your stools are lighter (whitish) in color.

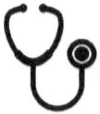 ## KIDNEY STONES

Acute spasmodic pain (excruciating, severe pain) that starts in your back (loin or kidney area), and seems to travel around the side of your abdomen to your groin may be a kidney stone.

This pain is called renal colic because it is a severe pain in the loin that comes and goes, and must be treated as an emergency.

You may have noticed your urine to be dark, or have passed blood mixed with urine.

The pain often goes when the stone is passed. Sometimes the stone cannot be passed, and you may need to have the stone broken into small pieces at the local hospital.

Analgesics and ibuprofen may not help, but antispasmodics can help to ease this pain.

Please go to hospital if you are passing blood with urine (haematuria).

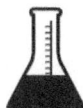
KNEE PAIN

This is a very common symptom that must first be self-treated before consulting a doctor. Doctors will first offer the same treatment that a chemist would advise.

The common treatment is anti-inflammatory analgesics like nitrogen, brufen, voltarol, and diclofenac with or without Paracetamol. The main problem with this is gastritis – tummy pain. People with gastritis must consult a doctor.

A doctor will do tests and investigations, and refer you to orthopedics or a rheumatologist if the pain does not resolve with anti-inflammatory drugs.

Please do not stop the treatment as soon as you feel that the pain has gone, but continue for two to three days.

Physiotherapy and exercise when you have pain is not good for you, because the inflamed joint is very brittle and can take more harm. You should exercise or get physiotherapy only after you have taken treatment and the pain has eased.

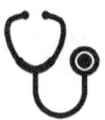
LEG PAIN AND SWELLING

Please check if the pain occurred after a fall or injury.

Severe pain and swelling of the leg, ankle or thigh soon after a fall indicates a fracture.

It is not easy to diagnose a fracture of the bone by clinical examination, so doctors will always request an X-Ray

You can use ice packs to help ease the pain.

Use sticks or splints to tie around the arm, using cloth or string to stabilize the arm or leg, before moving to hospital if the pain occurs when you move.

Severe pain can produce shock, so please leave the patient in a comfortable position. Even slight movement can trigger pain and produce shock.

The local temperature may increase, and the patient may be hyperventilating or very anxious.

Please do not offer them any drink. If the mouth is dry, try to moisturize the mouth. In hospital, doctors will organize an anaesthetic to help ease the pain or perform surgery. If the patient eats or drinks, the procedure will be delayed, so it is not a good idea to drink or eat but rather to remain starved.

You can also take Paracetamol and/or Non-Steroid Anti-Inflammatory Analgesics (NSAID), like nurofen or brufen. Please note that NSAIDs can irritate the stomach and cause stomach pain. Please DO NOT TAKE NSAIDs if you are allergic and/or know it can upset your tummy. Some people would also develop severe diarrhoea, and vomit blood, and so must not take this drug.

If the problem is in the neck and back, please check the information specific to those organs.

Please go to A&E in a hospital, because the doctor will need an X-Ray to rule out fractures or dislocations.

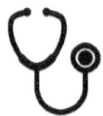 LEGS NOT MOVING

Babies, infants and children can suffer from a hip problem that makes them not move their legs.

This could spring from a congenitally dislocated hip, Perthes disease, osteoarthritis, rheumatoid arthritis, rheumatic fever, infection and/or traumatic damage. Fractures are not very rare.

Toddlers are notorious for often falling and hurting themselves. If the child is hyperactive, autistic, or inquisitive, he or she will run around the house or garden, and so it is difficult to be vigilant.

After a fall, the majority of these kids do not cry, because they have an adrenal surge that prevents them from experiencing pain. A few hours after the fall, they may stop moving their arms, or cry as pain starts kicking in.

Some parents may notice swelling, or identify localized pain in the shoulder, arm, elbow or wrist.

This can also happen a few days after the child develops a sore throat caused by a streptococcus infection. This was a common problem, known as "Rheumatic Fever" in the past, but declined after Penicillin became available. The antibodies produced to fight infection suddenly start attacking the joints and heart. Please consult a doctor and make sure to remind him or her about rheumatic fever. We anticipate that this infection may return soon.

Joint pain in children is not rare, and diagnosis depends on the root cause.

It is either poly-articular (multiple joints), mono-articular (one joint), fleeting arthritis, migrating arthritis (spreading from one joint to another or jumping from one joint to another).

Please consult a paediatrician to decide which specialist can help manage this problem. This may be a Rheumatologist or an Orthopedician.

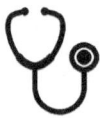# LIGHT HURTS CHILDS EYE

The diagnosis of this symptom requires proper clinical examination, and may require investigations.

Doctors will only treat this symptom after ruling out serious illnesses, so you must consult a doctor.

This is typically a symptom of meningitis but can also occur in allergic conjunctivitis. The only way we can differentiate these two is by clinical examination, so you must go to hospital and not wait to consult a GP.

Please do not panic, but go to A&E if you cannot get an appointment, or you cannot speak to or consult a doctor.

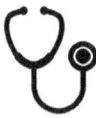# LIPS ARE BLUE

This is an emergency problem.

This symptom is most commonly associated with heart or lung problems.

Please do not waste time trying to find information, please go to hospital.

This is what we call "Central Cyanosis" indicating that blood is not getting enough oxygen and so is turning blue.

Please do not waste time, but call an ambulance and go to hospital now.

The doctors will examine the patient to differentiate between heart, lungs, and circulation problems.

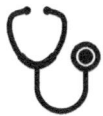 ## LOSS OF APPETITE

This is a very vague symptom, and there are not many illnesses or diseases associated with this symptom.

Depression, stress, viral infections, and psychological problems are said to be associated with a lack of appetite.

Patients with cancer on chemotherapy, an elderly person with dementia, or someone who has been on controlled drugs can experience this problem.

Doctors must investigate to identify the cause, and will check the blood to see if the person is anaemic, diabetic, or has some other metabolic disorder.

This is not an emergency, so please book an appointment to consult a doctor or nurse.

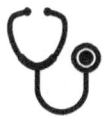 ## LOSS OF CONCENTRATION

Children with Autism, Attention Deficit Hyper Activity syndrome (ADHD), Dyslexia, and other learning disability disorders cannot concentrate.

Some mothers of toddlers or teenagers often label them as not listening or concentrating. This is likely to be a temporary stage, due to hyperactivity or hormonal changes. It is difficult to offer advice or treatment. These children often sleep less, so may also have mood swings and be irritable.

Adults on drugs for epilepsy, sedated, diabetic, and even on drugs like statin can experience reduced concentration. Drug abuse and alcoholism must be ruled out.

Please look for signs of depression, anxiety and other mental illnesses.

You will need to consult a doctor or nurse.

 ## LUMP – RED HOT PAINFUL

This is likely to be an abscess.

The diagnosis of this symptom requires proper clinical examination, and may require investigation.

The abscess must be drained and treated with antibiotics.

The problem doctors will have is to choose the right antibiotic, because almost all bacteria that produce an abscess are now resistant to treatment.

The worst thing you can do is to take low dose antibiotics, because the bacteria which are not yet resistant to treatment will soon learn to thrive despite antibiotics if they are exposed to a low dose only.

If the abscess is not treated early, the bacteria will enter the blood stream, spread all over the body and kill.

Doctors will only treat this symptom after ruling out serious illnesses so you must consult a DOCTOR.

Please do not panic, but go to A&E if you cannot get an appointment or you cannot speak to or consult a doctor.

 ## LUMP IN ANAL REGION

A common cause of a lump is hemorrhoids.

This is a painless, soft lump that may occasionally bleed during bowel movements. You might notice small amounts of bright red blood on your toilet tissue or in the toilet bowl.

Itching or irritation in your anal region is common if you are a smoker.

Hemorrhoids may be internal. These hemorrhoids lie inside the rectum, so you don't feel the lump but may notice bleeding, or have pain, discomfort, or develop constipation. Straining or irritation when passing stool can damage a hemorrhoid's delicate surface and cause it to bleed.

Occasionally, straining can push an internal hemorrhoid through the anal opening. This is known as a protruding or prolapsed hemorrhoid, and can cause pain and irritation.

External hemorrhoids are under the skin around your anus. When irritated, external hemorrhoids can itch or bleed.

Sometimes blood may pool in an external hemorrhoid and form a clot (thrombus), resulting in severe pain, swelling and inflammation.

Bleeding during bowel movements is the most common sign of hemorrhoids. But rectal bleeding can occur with other diseases.

If you have symptoms like bleeding, pain, changing bowel habits (constipation and diarrhoea), passing black, tarry, or maroon stools, blood clots, or blood mixed in with the stool, please consult your doctor immediately.

Go to hospital if you experience large amounts of rectal bleeding, light-headedness, dizziness or faintness.

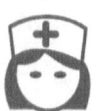 ## LUMP IN GROIN

This is a very common problem.

If the lump in the inguinal region (junction of thigh and abdomen) is painless and mobile, it is likely to be a lymph node.

If the lump is painful, or red and hot, then you have an abscess. This must be drained using a needle, or excised if it is loculated and large. Antibiotic treatment is now becoming problematic, as the bacteria causing the abscess are resistant to almost all antibiotics.

If the lymph node is matted, fixed, and not mobile, this could be a sign of tuberculosis and other infections.

Blood disorders and lymphomas also enlarge the lymph nodes.

You must consult a doctor or a nurse.

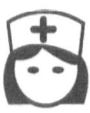 **LUMP ON EYE LID**

This is most likely to be a sty if it is associated with pain.

This small painful lump appears on the edge of the eyelid and gradually become bigger. It usually discharges spontaneously.

Chloromycetin drops and ointment applied to the lid margins should help.

If the sty is pointing, remove the lash to allow it to drain smoothly.

If styes are occurring regularly, please consult a doctor and find out why. You may need to be tested for diabetes.

Using hot water can help to ease the pain, and helps the sty to open and discharge its secretions

A chalazion (meibomian cyst) is a painless cyst in the eyelids, which may become painful if infected.

If infected, it is worth trying Chloromycetin ointment. Some chalazions will resolve spontaneously. If it is not resolving or uninfected, surgical curettage may be needed.

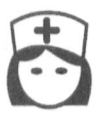 **MEASLES**

Children are most vulnerable to this highly contagious viral infection. With the MMR vaccination this is now very rare in the UK.

Symptoms usually develop in a well-established order: a mild to severe temperature of around 39°c/102.2°F, tiredness and general fatigue, a poor appetite, running nose and sneezing, irritable dry cough, red eyes, and sensitivity to light.

Tiny white spots appear in the mouth and throat, and a blotchy red rash starts behind the ears, spreads to the face, and then to the rest of the body, and lasts for up to seven days.

It takes around 10 to 12 days for the virus to make its presence felt after infection from another child. Physical contact, sneezing, and contact with clothing contaminated by nasal secretions all help to spread this infection.

Although immunization rates are now very high you should isolate your child from other children if you think they may be infected. Immunized children and those who have already caught Measles are virtually immune.

Meningitis and pneumonia are rare but can be serious secondary complications.

More commonly, the eyes and ears develop a secondary infection, which may need antibiotics from your doctor.

Once the rash starts, it is a matter of treating the symptoms.

Check the child's temperature. Use Paracetamol suspensions (e.g., Calpol) for fever, aches and pains.

Reducing sunlight or electric light in the room can help with the light sensitivity.

Use a ball of damp cotton wool to clean away any crustiness around the eyes.

Cough medicines are of little value, but do ease ticklish throats. Try placing a bowl of water in the room.

Avoid dehydration. Feverish small children rapidly lose water. It also makes a cough worse.

Ideally, you should keep your child away from others for at least 7 days after the start of the rash.

After four days the child usually feels better.

Protect your child against Measles – ensure that they are vaccinated with the MMR vaccination.

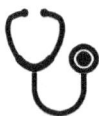 ## MEMORY LOSS

Everyone forgets things at some time, but if this becomes a regular problem and your quality of life is deteriorating as a result, you need help.

Mild cognitive impairment is a notable change in thinking skills that is limited for the most part, to a narrow set of problems, such as impairment only in memory.

Changes in concentration, attention, or mental quickness may also be observed. Mild cognitive impairment generally doesn't prevent a person from carrying out everyday tasks and being socially engaged.

Researchers and physicians are still learning much about mild cognitive impairment.

An elderly person with dementia or Alzheimer's disease, and epileptics and diabetics can develop this problem. Some drugs are also said to produce temporary memory loss.

Some degree of memory problems, as well as a modest decline in other thinking skills, is a fairly common part of aging. There's a difference, however, between normal changes in memory and the type of memory loss associated with Alzheimer's disease and related disorders. And some memory problems are the result of treatable conditions.

If you're experiencing memory problems, talk to your doctor to get a timely diagnosis and appropriate care.

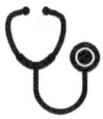 ## MENINGITIS

This is a rare illness that is well known all over the world.

It causes inflammation of the brain lining which can be fatal.

Unfortunately, the symptoms can be easily mistaken for flu or a bad cold. Worse still, it is more difficult to be certain with babies and young children. If you are not sure, you must call 111.

Hib immunization has reduced the number of people suffering from some types of meningitis or septicaemia.

Symptoms in babies under 2 years old: the babies can be difficult to wake, their cry may be high pitched and different from normal; they may vomit repeatedly, and not just after feeds; may refuse feeds, either from the bottle, the breast, or by spoon. Their skin may appear pale or blotchy, possibly with a red/purple rash, which does not fade when you press a tumbler glass or a finger against the rash.

The soft spot on top of your baby's head (the fontanels) may be tight or bulging.

The baby may seem irritable and dislike being handled.

The baby's body may be floppy, or else stiff with jerky movements. Remember that a fever may not be present in the early stages.

Older children may have slightly different symptoms:

A constant generalized headache, a high temperature, although their hands and feet may be cold, vomiting, drowsiness, confusion, and sensitivity to bright lights, daylight, or even the TV.

Neck stiffness – moving their chin to their chest will be very painful at the back of the neck.

A rash of red or purple spots or bruises, which does not fade when you press a tumbler glass or a finger against the rash. The rash may not be present in the early stages.

Other, rarer symptoms: Joint or muscle pain, rapid breathing, stomach pain, sometimes with diarrhoea.

Symptoms can appear in any order and not everyone gets all of the symptoms.

There are different types of meningitis, which can be caused by either bacteria or viruses.

A vaccination programme has now started for meningitis C for children and young people up to 17 years of age. Some forms of meningitis do not, as yet, have a vaccination, so the disease can still occur.

Note that people who have been in contact with someone who has had meningitis should contact a close relative of the patient to find out any instructions (from the hospital or the Director of Public Health) that they may have been given regarding antibiotics. Otherwise your doctor will be able to give you appropriate advice. Only those who have been in very close contact with the infected person are given antibiotics and vaccinations in response.

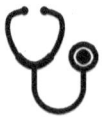

MERS, Middle East Respiratory Syndrome

MERS (Middle East Respiratory Syndrome) is a severe, pneumonia-like respiratory disease caused by a virus. It is different from SARS, because MERS is caused by another subtype of the virus. Pneumonia is a general term for an inflammation of the air sacs of the lungs caused by an infection or chemical. With pneumonia, the lungs fill with fluid, which interferes with their ability to transfer oxygen to the blood. MERS is known as an atypical pneumonia because it is not caused by the usual bacteria or viruses. MERS is typically associated with a high fever (over 38°C or 100.4°F), cough, severe shortness of breath, and diarrhoea. The infection is thought to be spread by close contact with an infected person. A virus called coronavirus is the cause of MERS. There are many kinds of coronavirus, some of which cause the common cold. The MERS coronavirus (MERS-CoV) is a new variant that was discovered in 2012 in the Middle Eastern region. How MERS spreads is not completely understood, but experts believe that the main way it spreads is through close contact with an infected person (by caring for or living with the person, or having direct contact with their respiratory secretions and body fluids). The people who have been infected by MERS have all been in a health care facility or among close family members. MERS is different from SARS. Most importantly, the MERS virus does not appear to be as easily spread between people, whereas the SARS virus spreads very easily.

PLEASE CONTACT AN ISOLATION HOSPITAL OR CALL THE EMERGENCY MERS HELPLINE. DO NOT GO TO A HOSPITAL OR CLINIC. THE ISOLATION UNIT WILL SEND DOCTORS AND AN AMBULANCE TO HELP ISOLATE YOU

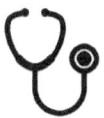 **MIGRAINE**

Migraines are a common illness that is often not diagnosed by a doctor because the illness runs in the family.

Visual patterns such as chequer boards or spots are often a warning of an impending attack. These can be quite debilitating, making the person sick and unable to concentrate.

The exact cause is still not known, although there is some connection with the blood vessels of the skull.

Certain foods appear to trigger migraines. Red wine, particularly Chianti, blue cheeses, and chocolate are all culprits.

Stress, the weather and even hormonal changes have been known to increase the suffering.

Avoid trigger foods such as red wine or blue cheese.

The greatest danger from headaches is missing something more serious than the expected causes. Irritability increases, along with a shorter fuse. There is a greater risk of having an accident, as well as a risk of overdosing on Paracetamol.

Please make sure you check and monitor your blood pressure.

Light can hurt the eyes, and lying in a darkened room helps for some people, although modern thought is to avoid such isolation and instead get on with 'normal' life.

The attack can last anywhere from minutes to days. There are treatments available from your doctor, which may reduce or even prevent a full-blown migraine attack. Anti-inflammatory drugs (e.g., ibuprofen) can help ease the pain, and are generally better than simple analgesics.

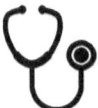 MISCARRAIGE

Miscarriage is the spontaneous loss of a pregnancy before the 20th week. Most miscarriages occur before 12 weeks of pregnancy.

About 10 to 20 percent of known pregnancies end in miscarriage. But the actual number is probably much higher, because many miscarriages occur so early in pregnancy that a woman doesn't even know she's pregnant when it happens.

Miscarriage is a somewhat loaded term — possibly suggesting that something was amiss in the carrying of the pregnancy. This is rarely true. Most miscarriages occur because the foetus is not developing normally. However, because these abnormalities are rarely understood, it's often difficult to determine what causes them.

Miscarriage is a relatively common experience — but that doesn't make it any easier. Take a step towards emotional healing by seeking to understand what can cause a miscarriage, what increases the risk, and what medical care might be needed.

If you are seeing mild bleeding or spotting, have cramping pain in your abdomen or lower back, or have some watery fluid or tissue passing from your vagina, please do not panic, because most women who experience vaginal spotting or bleeding in the first trimester go on to have successful pregnancies.

Passing clots and foetal products is common but may not be obvious. Some women are not aware of the pregnancy and often do not notice this one-off painless event, which often lasts for a day or two.

This can be a traumatic period for some, so please do call and speak to your doctor.

Sexually active women who have missed periods must get a pregnancy test, because they may have some blood problem which will need to be identified, and often need to be treated after abortion or childbirth.

Please go to an antenatal clinic in the hospital, or speak to your doctor.

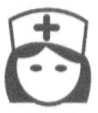 **MUMPS**

Mumps is characterized by swelling or pain in the parotid glands and sub-mandibular area (in front of the ears and neck), a dry mouth, worse pain on swallowing or chewing, a fever (high to very high), malaise, headache, drowsiness, vomiting, abdominal (tummy)

pain, and photophobia: cannot stand bright light. This may also be associated with testicular pain.

The incubation period of mumps is 12–28 days. The patient is infectious from 3 days prior to the swelling until 7 days after it resolves.

This was once a common disease in children, which became very rare following the introduction of the mumps vaccination. Unfortunately, this disease is likely to return, as viruses and bacteria are becoming resistant to treatment and learning to overcome immunity.

There may be mild prodromal symptoms prior to the swelling of the salivary glands. Parotid glands (below the ears) are nearly always affected.

Women must get a pregnancy test, as this infection can damage the foetus.

Most cases are without serious consequence, but complications include orchitis, pancreatitis, viral meningitis, and the risk of miscarriage between 12 and 16 weeks' gestation.

Paracetamol or ibuprofen help reduce the pain and fever, and you should maintain a high fluid intake.

Avoid acidic fruit juices, because it may increase the pain and should be avoided.

Go to hospital if:

There is abdominal pain in the left side radiating to back: Pancreatitis caused by infected pancreases

Testicular pain is present: Orchitis is rare before puberty, usually unilateral and rarely, if ever, causes infertility.

Oophoritis – infected ovaries. If you are pregnant, give this special attention.

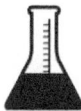 # NAPPY RASH

Rashes in the nappy area are common, but can be reduced in severity or avoided completely. Frequent nappy changes, and leaving nappies off to provide exposure to air for part of the day will prevent nappy rash occurring.

If you are keen to apply nappy cream when you are using an over dry nappy, please use the cream or ointment when the child is naked.

This rash is usually red, not raised and confined to the nappy area.

It is caused by the irritating effect of urine and bowel motions. If they are cleaned away quickly enough, nappy rash will not appear. As far as is possible, you should change each nappy quickly following soiling.

Remember that urine can be every bit as irritating as faeces.

Avoid disposable wipes containing alcohol or moisturizing chemicals. Instead use plenty of warm water. As much as is practical, leave the nappy off, particularly any plastic pants.

Dry, cool skin rarely forms a nappy rash.

Reusable nappies should be washed as directed by the manufacturer.

Avoid caustic household detergents when washing a reusable nappy.

An angry red rash, which does not respond to treatment or extends beyond the nappy area, may be a fungal infection (Candida). You will need to treat this with an antifungal cream and an oral antifungal agent as it often starts in the mouth.

Promptly treat any rash that appears with ointment from your pharmacist. Please do not use any cream if you are regularly using "Dry Nappies."

If the rash is present in the crease between the thigh and abdomen, the child will need an antifungal cream and treatment for oral thrush.

Avoid talcum powder generally, as it can cake badly and cause even more irritation.

If the rash is severe or resistant, it may be a candida infection.

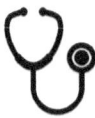 ## NAUSEA

Nausea is a sensation of uneasiness and discomfort in the upper stomach (left upper aspect of abdomen). This is often followed by the involuntary urge to vomit.

You can be nauseous but never vomit. This occurs with allergies, migraines, and vertigo.

The most common cause of nausea and vomiting is food poisoning. The key is to differentiate between chemical, bacterial and viral infections. If the nausea, followed by vomiting occurs within six hours of consuming some food, it is rated as chemical poisoning. Drugs, gastritis which follows alcohol consumption, infections, and also problems in the brain and ears can produce nausea. Gastroenteritis is diagnosed if this symptom is associated with diarrhoea. The diagnosis of this symptom requires proper clinical examination and may require investigation. Doctors will only treat this symptom after ruling out serious illnesses so please consult a DOCTOR. Please do not panic, but go to A&E or the ER if you cannot get an appointment, or you cannot speak to or consult a doctor.

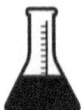 ## NECK PAIN

This is a common complaint, but not one that is usually serious.

Neck muscles can be strained from poor posture when sleeping, or from sitting during work leaning over your computer or hunching over your workbench. Osteoarthritis is also a common cause of neck pain.

Seek medical care if your neck pain is accompanied by numbness or loss of strength in your arms or hands, or if you have shooting pains into your shoulder or down your arm.

You may find it hard to move your neck and so hold your head in one place for long periods, such as when driving or working at a computer.

Muscle tightness and spasms lead to a decreased ability to move your head, and you may develop a headache.

Your neck is flexible, and supports the weight of your head, so it can be vulnerable to injuries and conditions that cause pain and restrict motion. Common causes are muscle strains, osteoarthritis, nerve compression, trauma, road traffic accidents, injuries, rheumatoid arthritis, and meningitis.

See your doctor if severe neck pain results from an injury, such as a motor vehicle accident, a diving accident, or a fall.

Contact a doctor if your neck pain is severe, persists for several days without relief, or you experience pain radiating down your arms or legs.

If associated with headache, numbness, weakness or tingling, contact a doctor immediately.

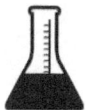 **NETTLE RASH**

Hives are small, often itchy, raised, red spots, which you can feel, and are rarely serious unless combined with any breathing problems.

The rash will usually disappear in a few hours without any treatment.

It is most often caused by certain foods and plants (e.g., nettles), but may also be caused by a viral infection.

A pharmacist may be able to recommend a cream or medicine that could provide some relief.

If the rash is severe and associated with breathing difficulties; or if there is any shortness of breath, dial 999.

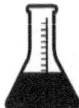 **NO FEVER**

Please use this if you have other symptoms that are not associated with increased body temperature.

This is very important information to help doctors differentiate some common illnesses.

If you are breathless and coughing but your body temperature is not increased, the cause could be asthma or foreign body aspiration.

If you have a rash that comes and goes and you have swollen lips, then the diagnosis is likely to be an urticarial or allergic rash.

You may have an increased heart rate associated with or without fever if you have a high body metabolic rate, as seen with an overactive thyroid, beriberi, anaemia, exercise, anxiety, excitement, and having sex.

Your body temperature and heart rate will always increase if you have bacterial or viral infections. Some metabolic or hormonal problems will often increase at the same time, and you may feel that the heart is beating faster.

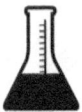 **NO OTHER SYMPTOM**

Please note MAYA will only be useful to you and offer the right advice if you have two + No Fever or three symptoms.

We have used this tool to help us diagnose illnesses for almost thirty years, and have not missed critical signs or made clinical diagnostic errors.

Doctors who do not listen to the patient, identify three associated symptoms, and who offer leading questions have made diagnostic errors.

MAYA does not offer leading questions, but we know you will choose the right symptom and get the correct information you need.

If you have only one symptom, please consult your own doctors as soon as possible, or continue searching for information on the Internet.

If you insist on identifying the cause of one symptom, you will be clinically examined, have investigations, and may be hospitalized for procedures that are not required.

Doctors will only treat patients when they have identified the combination of symptoms that suggest infection, infestation or illness (disease). When the combination of symptoms is not related to one another, they label this as a Syndrome.

Well-trained and experienced doctors will offer advice or treatment after ruling out common serious illnesses.

Please do not panic, but go to A&E or the ER if you cannot get an appointment or you cannot speak to or consult a doctor.

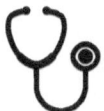 **NOISY BREATHING**

This is a vague symptom that sounds like your nose is blocked, or you may hear a grunting noise when breathing.

If the noise is coming from the nose, it is usually prolonged, but the short grunts come from the chest and it seems like the person is struggling to breathe.

They may or may not be cyanosed.

Babies grunt when they have chest infections like pneumonia. The body temperature in these cases is mild-moderate, and the baby will be breathless. They look anxious, and are often alert.

Most patients with breathlessness and grunt will need hospital treatment, because they will require IV antibiotics.

If not treated early, this condition will deteriorate. Please call 999 and go to the hospital. If the sound is musical, and/or sounds like wheezing, check out "asthma" and "cough with wheezing."

Other sounds are due to problems in the throat like a stridor or due to a floppy larynx (voice box).

Specialists in hospital usually do the diagnosing of this symptom.

Please consult a doctor, and organize a referral to a specialist.

If the other symptoms associated with this illness are RED, please go to the ER or A&E in a hospital

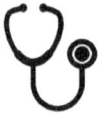 **NOSE BLEEDING**

Common causes of this are a blood vessel bursting during sneezing, allergies or spontaneously due to deficiencies.

Bleeding occurs when the clotting mechanism has gone wrong or the blood has low platelets but these are very rare causes and can only be diagnosed after blood test.

Specialists must investigate recurrent bleeds in the hospital.

Diagnosis of this symptom requires a proper clinical examination and blood tests, and may require other investigations.

Doctors will first check your blood pressure, and only treat the symptom after ruling out serious illnesses.

Please do not panic, but try to pinch your nose for 5 to 10 minutes, and make sure the bleeding stops. If it does not, go to A&E or the ER.

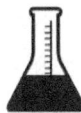 ## NOSE BLOCKED

The most common cause of this symptom is allergies.

The irritation of allergens (dust, pollens or chemicals) will produce inflammation in the nose, resulting in the swelling of mucous membrane inside the nostril. This swelling will block the passage.

You may have a deviated nasal septum (DNS), but an operation will only help you for some time, because the septum will grow back and block the passage again.

If one nasal passage is getting blocked on and off, you may have DNS, and allergic irritation will usually block one nostril more than the other.

If the symptom is often chronic, is not associated with fever, and is associated with excessive sneezing and a runny nose, treat this as hay fever.

The most common cause of blocked nostrils is rhinitis, hay fever, or allergic irritants (smoke, perfume, etc.).

Virus or bacterial infection in the sinuses, throat, nose and ears can also produce the same symptom.

Xylometazoline hydrochloride nasal spray will help to open up and clear nasal passages by reducing nasal mucosal thickening and returning swollen blood vessels to their normal size. This drug provides up to 10 hours of relief in as little as 2 minutes. Please note that this drug will make the symptom worse if you continue using it for more than three to five days.

If the problem is chronic, please do not assume you have the common cold.

Please read all about "rhinitis" and get the correct treatment.

Please note that there is no drug that cures this, only those that offer symptomatic treatment – your symptoms will be relieved only while you use the nasal spray.

If this symptom exists for long time, the chances of getting a bacterial infection are high and so you will need antibiotics.

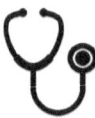 ## NUMBNESS

This is a sign of nerve problems, and must be seen by a doctor.

You are likely to have this as a single symptom, and if so, please consult a neurologist.

Some areas of skin in our body can have become numb because you have had an injury or infected skin there that has killed the nerve endings.

 ## OFFENSIVE DISCHARGE

Chronic pelvic disease is common in sexually active women.

Please check for foreign bodies like retained product or parts of a tampon.

If this symptom is associated with feeling hot and cold, you must treat this as an emergency, and go to hospital for investigation and antibiotic treatment.

GO TO A GUM (Genitourinary clinic) or STD (Sexually Transmitted Disease) walk-in-clinic.

 ## PAINFUL PERIODS

This is a common problem, known as dysmenorrhoea.

You must start taking brufen or mefanamic acid (Non-Steroidal Anti-inflammatory tablet) 2–3 days before the day you are expecting your period, and then continue taking this drug during menstruation.

Please do not take NSAIDs if you are suffering from gastritis, recurrent abdominal pain, or are a person who is allergic. Stop treatment as soon as the period ends.

If this does not improve, then make an appointment with a family planning clinic to see if taking contraceptive pills can help.

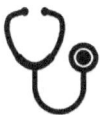 **PAIN IN ABDOMEN**

Other popular terms for abdominal pain include tummy pain, tummy ache, stomach ache, stomach pain, gut ache, and belly ache. Pain that originates between the chest and the pelvis is labeled as tummy pain or stomach ache, stomach pain, gut ache, bellyache and gut rot.

The abdomen is that part of your body which is below your ribs, and above your hips. Some people call it the trunk, tummy, belly, or gut.

Pain that you feel here is usually linked to a problem in your gut, but you may be experiencing referred pain from problems existing in your chest or groin.

Pain in the abdomen (tummy pain) is a very common symptom that can be very difficult for doctors to diagnose, and frustrating for affected patients.

Pain that is severe, or doesn't settle quickly, must be examined and managed only by a doctor in the hospital. If not, the chances of long-term complications are very high.

This is one symptom that can catch many doctors by surprise, because they forget to examine the chest, abdomen, and groin areas to rule out referred pain. If you are not happy with the doctors or nurses, and feel that they have not listened, or have offered treatment or advice without carrying out a clinical examination of the chest, groin, and abdomen, please consult another doctor. Common causes of abdominal pain are gastritis, gastro-enteritis, trapped wind, and diarrhoea.

If the symptoms are not resolved, you must consult a specialist and not waste time.

Please make sure you do not drink or eat, if the symptoms associated suggest you to go to hospital as an emergency.

If you have recently eaten, doctors will not be able to perform surgical procedures if they need to.

Different types of pain you may feel are: sharp or stabbing, crimpy, spasmodic, colicky, or a general dull ache. Colicky pain is sharp, spasmodic (on and off), and gradually becoming worse.

Doctors may also be interested in whether the pain seems to be radiating (travelling) in a certain direction.

Having this information, and putting it together with other information (such as whether you have been vomiting, or had diarrhoea, etc.), will help the doctor work out what is wrong.

Pain that comes on suddenly may be called acute. Longer-standing pain is called chronic.

Common causes of abdominal pain are: indigestion, wind, constipation, Irritable Bowel Syndrome, appendicitis, kidney stones, a urine infection, pelvic inflammatory disease, gall stones, period pain, food poisoning, stomach and duodenal ulcers, and Crohn's disease.

You may recognize your type of pain from the descriptions here. However, if you have a pain that is not going away quickly (within a few hours), or that you cannot cope with, you must go to a hospital, and not wait for an appointment to consult a GP.

Delays in diagnosis and getting the right treatment often result in short-term and long-term complications.

DO NOT PANIC, but go to A&E if you cannot get an appointment or you cannot speak to or consult a doctor.

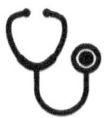

PAIN AND LUMP IN THROAT

This is often associated with pharyngitis or problems with the vocal cords. If you have fever, then the most likely cause is pharyngitis.

You need specific antibiotics, and so may require investigation and referral to a specialist.

An abscess in the throat known as quincy can also alter the voice. This problem may require hospital treatment.

The diagnosis of this symptom requires proper clinical examination, and may require investigation.

Doctors will only treat this symptom after ruling out serious illnesses so you must consult a DOCTOR.

Please do not panic, but go to A&E or the ER if you cannot get an appointment, or you cannot speak to or consult a doctor.

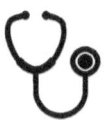

PAIN AND SWELLING AFTER A FALL

Severe pain and swelling of the hands, leg, ankle, arms, wrist, thigh, or face soon after a fall indicates a fracture.

It is not easy to diagnose a fracture of the bone by clinical examination, so doctors will always request an X-Ray

You can use ice packs to help ease the pain.

Use sticks or splints to tie around the arm, using cloth or string to stabilize the arm or leg, before moving to hospital if the pain occurs when you move.

Severe pain can produce shock, so please leave the patient in a comfortable position. Even slight movement can trigger pain and produce shock.

The local temperature may increase, and the patient may be hyperventilating or very anxious.

Please do not offer them any drink. If the mouth is dry, try to moisturize the mouth. In hospital, doctors will organize an anaesthetic to help ease the pain or perform surgery. If the patient eats or drinks, the procedure will be delayed, so it is not a good idea to drink or eat but rather to remain starved.

You can also take Paracetamol and/or non-steroidal Anti-Inflammatory Analgesics (NSAID), like nurofen or brufen. Please note that NSAIDs can irritate the stomach and cause stomach pain. Please DO NOT TAKE NSAIDs if you are allergic and/or know it can upset your tummy. Some people would also develop severe diarrhoea, and vomit blood, and so must not take this drug.

If the problem is in the neck and back, please check the information specific to those organs.

Please go to A&E in a hospital, because the doctor will need an X-Ray to rule out fractures or dislocations.

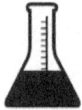 PAIN IN BOTH EARS

In the case of a viral infection, both ears will have effusion and there will be pain in both ears.

Wax will not be present in the ear if the eardrum is inflamed.

If the doctors or nurses say you have mild wax and the drum looks red, this is unlikely to be true. If the eardrum is inflamed, wax will melt and you may have some turbid discharge.

Please do not use cotton buds to clear the block, because the buds will push the soft melting wax inside, and the pain may increase.

A viral infection will not be killed by antibiotics, but they will kill healthy bacteria and encourage resistant strains to colonize your body.

Please note that doctors must use a "pneumatic otoscope" and check pressure in the middle ear to diagnose otitis media (an ear infection) before prescribing antibiotics.

Please read about pneumatic otoscopy on the Internet, and educate your doctor about the importance of making the right diagnosis before prescribing antibiotics.

Using low dose antibiotics or prescribing antibiotic eardrops will help bacteria to develop resistance.

Wrong diagnoses and mistreatment of bacterial infections in the ear can result in complications like perforation or septicaemia.

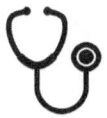 **PAIN IN ONE EAR**

The common cause of pain in one ear is likely to be impacted wax, but bacterial infections can also start in one ear and then spread to the other ear.

Virus infections that do not require antibiotics often occur in both ears.

Check the associated symptoms to help differentiate bacterial and viral infections, and consult a nurse to get the ear examined properly.

Please note that doctors must use a "pneumatic otoscope" and check pressure in the middle ear to diagnose otitis media (an ear infection) before prescribing antibiotics.

Please read about pneumatic otoscopy on the Internet, and educate your doctor about the importance of making the right diagnosis before prescribing antibiotics.

Using low dose antibiotics or prescribing antibiotic eardrops will help bacteria to develop resistance.

Wrong diagnoses and mistreatment of bacterial infections in the ear can result in complications like perforation or septicaemia.

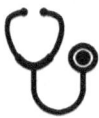 PAIN IN TESTES

A doctor must see pain in or around one or both testicles in the scrotum as an emergency.

Sometimes testicle pain actually originates from somewhere else in the groin or abdomen, and is felt in one or both testicles (referred pain).

Torsion of testes is common in children but children may present with other symptoms like abdominal pain, vomiting, an irritable cry, etc., and so this may be missed.

The testicles are very sensitive, and even a minor injury can cause testicle pain or discomfort. Testicle pain may arise from within the testicle itself, or from the coiled tube and supporting tissue behind the testicle (epididymis).

Sometimes, what seems to be testicle pain is caused by a problem that starts in the groin, the abdomen, or somewhere else (kidney stones and some hernias may cause testicle pain).

The cause of testicle pain can't always be identified.

Please consult a doctor as an emergency.

 **PAIN IN VAGINA**

This is commonly the result of dyspareunia.

Pain in the vagina is common during intercourse, at entry, or with deep thrusting.

Emotional factors can be associated with many types of painful intercourse.

A dry vagina (lack of secretion) can mean that there was not enough foreplay, insufficient lubrication, or low oestrogen levels (for example, after childbirth or during breast-feeding).

Drugs like antidepressants, blood pressure medications, sedatives, antihistamines, and certain birth control pills can contribute to this symptom.

It could also stem from injury, trauma or irritation, inflammation, infection, a skin disorder, vaginismus, congenital abnormalities, illnesses and conditions like endometriosis, pelvic inflammatory disease, uterine prolapse, an extroverted uterus, uterine fibroids, cystitis, irritable bowel syndrome, hemorrhoids, ovarian cysts, or the presence of a foreign body.

Psychological problems that may contribute include stress and stress stemming from past sexual abuse.

This is not an emergency, but if you are bleeding then go to hospital and consult a gynaecologist.

Please consult a doctor and get a proper internal examination.

Try using lubricants like KY Jelly if the problem is dryness. Consult a doctor, or contact Relate if this is connected to a relationship problem.

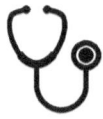 # PAIN IN VAGINA DURING AND AFTER SEX

Pain during or after sex has become a common problem. This is known as dyspareunia.

The major causes are stress, lack of foreplay, illness, infection, and other physical or psychological problems

If you are suffering from this problem, please speak to a doctor. They are used to this and will not be embarrassed.

Pain during sex can affect both men and women.

Tablets like Viagra and others are making sexual intercourse last longer. If the woman is not properly stimulated, the vagina can be dry, and mucosal tears can be traumatic.

Some women are allergic to latex and plastic materials.

Women can experience pain during or after sex, either in the vagina or deeper in the pelvis. Pain in the vagina could be caused by an infection like thrush, chlamydia, gonorrhoea, or genital herpes.

During the menopause, hormone levels can make your vagina dry (vaginitis).

Lack of sexual arousal and vaginismus occur because the muscles in or around the vagina shut tightly, making sex painful or impossible.

Genital irritation or allergic reactions can be caused by spermicides, latex condoms, or products such as soap and shampoo

Pain felt inside the pelvis can be caused by conditions such as pelvic inflammatory disease or endometriosis.

See your GP, or go to a sexual health GUM (genitourinary medicine) clinic.

Using KY jelly can help to ease the problem.

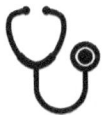 ## PAIN WORSE WHEN CLIMBING UP

This very common symptom is associated with knee pain.

People with congestive heart failure, chest problems, and pneumonia may also complain of this symptom.

Knee pain as you climb up the stairs is the first sign of arthritis.

Pain in the front of the knee is a common complaint at all ages, especially for women.

Most anterior knee pain is related to the patellofemoral joint and its musculature and ligament support.

It is two to seven times more prevalent in women than men.

It is estimated that up to 10 percent of all knee pain that accompanies aging is due to isolated patellofemoral arthritis. Because the exact source of pain can be difficult to isolate, and is often multifactorial, patellofemoral pain syndrome requires a careful diagnosis and proper management, to avoid unnecessary, ineffective, or potentially harmful treatments.

A common treatment is anti-inflammatory analgesics like nurofen, brufen, voltarol, and diclofenac with or without paracetamol. The main problem with this is gastritis – tummy pain.

A doctor will do tests, investigations and referral to orthopedics or rheumatologist if the pain does not resolve with anti-inflammatory drugs.

Do not stop the treatment as soon as you feel the pain has gone but continue for two to three days.

Physiotherapy and exercise when you have pain is not good because the inflamed joint is very brittle and can cause more harm.

You must exercise or get physio only after you have taken treatment and pain has eased.

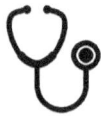 PAIN WORSE WHILE CLIMBING DOWN

This symptom must be examined and managed by doctors.

Please read the information in "Pain worse when climbing up."

This very common symptom is associated with knee pain.

People with congestive heart failure, chest problems, or pneumonia may also complain of this symptom.

The protective covering of the knee joint's surface is probably damaged, and the padding known as meniscus may be torn.

This is one symptom that must be managed by an orthopedic surgeon.

The common treatment is anti-inflammatory analgesics like nurofen, brufen, voltarol, and diclofenac with or without paracetamol. The main problem with this is gastritis – tummy pain. People with gastritis must consult a doctor.

A doctor will do tests and investigations, and refer you to orthopedics or a rheumatologist if the pain does not resolve with anti-inflammatory drugs.

Please do not stop the treatment as soon as you feel that the pain has gone, but continue for two to three days.

Physiotherapy and exercise when you have pain is not good for you, because the inflamed joint is very brittle and can take more harm. You must exercise or get physiotherapy only after you have taken treatment and the pain has eased.

You may require arthroscopy (a minor surgical procedure) to rule out meniscal tears and floaters in the knee joint.

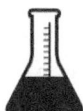 ## PAINFUL ANKLE

This is a very common symptom that can be managed with a chemist's help.

You must self-treat this symptom before consulting a doctor. Doctors will first offer the same treatment that a chemist would advise. The most common treatment is anti-inflammatory analgesics like nurofen, brufen, voltarol, and diclofenac with or without paracetamol. The main side effect of these is gastritis – tummy pain. People who have gastritis must consult a doctor.

A doctor will do tests, investigations, and refer you to orthopedics or a rheumatologist if the pain does not resolve with anti-inflammatory drugs. Please do not block an appointment in the surgery if you have not already taken the treatment as advised by a chemist.

Do not stop the treatment as soon as you feel the pain has gone but continue it for two to three more days. Physical therapy and exercise when you have pain is not good for you, because the inflamed joint is very brittle and can take more harm. You should exercise or get physiotherapy only after you have taken treatment and the pain has eased. If the problem is chronic, please consult a doctor.

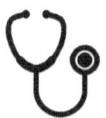 ## PAINFUL LUMP IN ANUS

A common cause of this kind of lump is thrombosis hemorrhoids. This is likely to present as a painful lump that may bleed during bowel movements. You might notice small amounts of bright red blood on your toilet tissue or in the toilet bowl, swelling around your anus, or a lump near your anus, which may be sensitive or painful.

Hemorrhoids may be internal or felt externally.

Internal hemorrhoids may start bleeding or produce pain and discomfort when you develop constipation. But any straining or irritation when passing a stool can damage a hemorrhoid's delicate surface and cause it to bleed.

Occasionally, straining can push an internal hemorrhoid through the anal opening. This is known as a protruding or prolapsed hemorrhoid, and can cause pain and irritation.

External hemorrhoids are under the skin around your anus. When irritated, external hemorrhoids can itch or bleed.

Sometimes blood may pool in an external hemorrhoid and form a clot (thrombus), resulting in severe pain, swelling and inflammation.

Bleeding during bowel movements is the most common sign of hemorrhoids. But rectal bleeding can occur with other diseases.

If you have symptoms like bleeding, pain, changing bowel habits (constipation and diarrhoea), passing black, tarry, or maroon stools, blood clots, or blood mixed in with the stool, please consult your doctor immediately.

Go to hospital if you experience large amounts of rectal bleeding, light-headedness, dizziness or faintness.

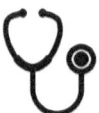 PALPITATIONS

With palpitations, you feel as if the heart is beating fast, fluttering or pounding.

Palpitations can be triggered by stress, exercise, excitement, medication or, rarely, a medical condition.

Palpitations are usually harmless. But this can occasionally be a symptom of a more serious heart condition, such as an irregular heartbeat (arrhythmia) that may require treatment.

You may feel as if the heart is skipping beats, fluttering, beating too fast, or working harder than usual.

Palpitations can be felt in your throat or neck, as well as in your chest.

They can occur even when you are resting, sleeping, sitting, standing or lying down.

The common causes of heart palpitations are strong emotional responses, stress or anxiety, strenuous exercise, caffeine, nicotine, and fever.

This symptom may also be connected to hormone changes associated with menstruation, pregnancy, or menopause, cold and cough medications that contain pseudoephedrine, a stimulant, and poor technique when using an asthma inhaler.

Please consult a doctor to rule out an overactive thyroid gland (hyperthyroidism), or an abnormal heart rhythm (arrhythmia). Arrhythmias may include very fast heart rates (tachycardia); unusually slow heart rates (bradycardia) or an irregular heart rhythm.

If you have a history of heart disease, and have frequent palpitations or have palpitations that worsen, talk to your doctor.

Treat this as an emergency if you also experience chest discomfort or pain, fainting, severe shortness of breath, or dizziness.

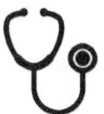 PASSING LESS URINE

Passing less urine more often is a common symptom to be seen when you have urinary tract infection.

There may be associated symptoms like fever which can help to confirm this diagnosis.

You will need a urine culture and microscopy. If blood and proteins are present in urine, the nitrate test is often positive. But if the infection is tested for early, this test may be negative. Please note that this test does not always confirm or rule out the presence of infection, and so must not be relied upon. Patients have developed serious septicaemia because they did not receive the right treatment early.

Please do not waste time before starting treatment if you have all the symptoms that suggest a urinary tract infection, but please make sure you have collected and sent a sample of urine off for testing (microscope and culture sensitivity) in the laboratory.

E.Coli is a common cause of this symptom, and we know the majority of its organisms are resistant to treatment. If symptoms like fever, and pain when passing urine are not better after taking three doses of antibiotics, please consult your doctor and get a urine test.

You must check the lab results before changing the antibiotics or getting admitted to hospital for intra-venous antibiotic treatment.

Please make sure that you get your blood pressure checked regularly.

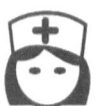 PASSING MORE URINE

This is common in elderly patients with heart failure, who are often taking water tablets that make them pass more urine.

This is not a common problem but can be associated with hormonal changes, salt and water abnormalities, infection, and kidney or heart problems.

If you are vomiting and/or have other symptoms that are red, you must go to a hospital and get the right treatment soon. Please treat this as an acute presentation of a serious illness that requires an emergency appointment.

Diabetes is one of the most common causes of this symptom, and it is often associated with excessive thirst.

If you are forcing yourself to drink excess water because someone told you to drink more water every day, then the problem is likely to be what we call psychogenic polyuria and polydipsia.

If you are not very ill, get a blood sugar test done in a local pharmacist. If the sugar levels are high, make an appointment and consult a nurse.

Please make sure that the doctor or nurse checks your blood pressure.

If you have other associated symptoms like vomiting, behavioral changes, weakness, loss of weight, pain when passing urine, or blood in your urine, please treat this as an emergency.

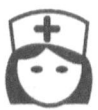 **PERIOD PAINS**

This is a common problem, and is known as dysmenorrhoea.

You must start taking brufen or mefanamic acid (Non-Steroidal Anti-inflammatory tablets) 2–3 days before the day you are expecting your period, and then continue taking this drug during menstruation.

Please do not take NSAIDs if you are suffering from gastritis, recurrent abdominal pain, or are a person who is allergic. Stop treatment as soon as the period ends.

If this does not improve, then make an appointment with a family planning clinic to see if taking contraceptive pills can help.

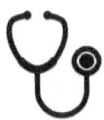 **PELVIC INFECTION**

The presenting symptom of a pelvic infection is often excessive, foul smelling vaginal discharge.

Pelvic inflammatory disease (PID), is an infection of the womb (uterus and or fallopian tubes).

Pain in the lower abdomen (pelvic area) is the most common symptom. It can range from mild to severe.

Pain and/or bleeding during sex can also occur.

Chlamydia, gonococcus, syphilis, staphylococcus, E. Coli and other bacteria can thrive in the womb, and will be difficult to treat. You must consult a gynaecologist or a sexually transmitted disease specialist in the genitourinary department (GUM Clinic) to identify the organisms involved and determine the antibiotic that is required.

This infection can be treated using the right antibiotics. If it is not, women can develop infertility, or have serious problems during pregnancy.

We anticipate that this will be a major problem in the future, because treatment resistant gonococcus, chlamydia, and syphilis are coming back with a vengeance.

Teenagers have become more sexually active in the last ten years. As a result, incidences of these infections have rapidly increased in the western world.

Please consult a gynaecologist, or go to a GUM clinic, because the long-term problems like infertility and other problems associated with PID will be difficult to manage.

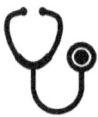 **PEPTIC ULCER**

Gastric ulcers affect the lining of the stomach, and are more common in people over 40 years old.

Prolonged use of high doses of steroids, perhaps for asthma or rheumatic conditions, can cause a gastric ulcer. Even relatively small doses of anti-inflammatory drugs such as ibuprofen or aspirin can lead to an ulcer in the stomach in people who are susceptible.

Duodenal ulcers, which are found lower down in the abdomen, are more common in men.

They heal more easily than the gastric variety, and usually develop just at the beginning of the duodenum.

The symptoms of peptic ulcers tend to overlap with other conditions, but a fairly general pattern is recognized.

Please consult a doctor to organize a breath test and blood tests to rule out H. Pylori infections.

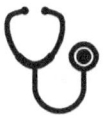 PERIODS IRREGULAR

In this symptom, periods, also known as menstruation, become irregular.

On an average, a woman gets her period every 21 to 35 days and it usually lasts about three to five days.

With menstrual cycle abnormality, the time between each period starts to alter. The woman will lose a greater or lesser quantity of blood in each cycle. The number of days that the period lasts also varies.

There are different names for different types of irregular periods.

Oligomenorrhea refers to infrequent periods, a condition in which the time between periods is typically 35 days or more. Women with Oligomenorrhea have fewer than six to eight periods a year.

Metrorrhagia refers to irregular, but still frequent periods.

Menometrorrhagia refers to longer or heavier periods that are irregular, but still frequent.

Amenorrhea refers to an absence of periods for at least three months.

Treatment depends on the cause of the irregularity, and your desire (or not) to have children in the future. Many different illnesses can cause irregular periods by changing the level of the hormones oestrogen and progesterone in the body.

This symptom is common in young girls going through puberty, and women during menopause will also have irregular periods.

Other common causes of irregular periods include: Polycystic ovaries, an intra-uterine device (IUD), oral contraception, excessive exercise, pregnancy, breast-feeding, an over active thyroid, fibroids, and uterus abnormalities.

Usually, no treatment is needed for irregular periods caused by puberty and the menopause unless they are excessive.

In other cases, the available courses of action would be to correct or treat the underlying disease, change oral contraceptive, engage in lifestyle management, hormone treatment, or surgery.

 PERIODS MISSED

The menstrual abnormality known as Amenorrhea refers to an absence of periods for at least three to six months.

On average, a woman gets her period every 21 to 35 days and usually lasts about three to five days.

Treatment depends on the cause and your desire (or not) to have children in the future.

This is not necessarily urgent unless you have pain, a fever, or discharge is present.

Please get a pregnancy test done by your chemist and consult a nurse in the local family planning clinic.

Many different illnesses can cause irregular periods by changing the level of the hormones oestrogen and progesterone in the body.

Irregularities are common in young girls going through puberty and women experiencing the menopause.

Other common causes of irregular or missed periods are an Intra-uterine device (IUD), oral contraception, excessive exercise, excessive weight loss, pregnancy, breast-feeding, a thyroid problem, fibroids or uterus abnormalities.

Identify the cause and seek treatment.

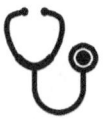 ## PHOTOPHOBIA

This is a common medical term meaning a fear of light. It is an abnormal intolerance to light, the fear of discomfort or pain to the eyes due to light exposure, or the presence of actual physical sensitivity of the eyes.

Common causes are allergic conjunctivitis and serious illnesses like meningitis. Other causes are migraines, headaches, cataracts, a brain injury, uveitis, blepharitis, coloboma, congenital abnormalities, corneal ulcers, conjunctivitis, injury, allergic conjunctivitis, or infections such as chalazion.

The cause and trigger factor must be identified before treatment is offered.

This can be caused due to conditions related to the eyes or nervous system, for example: too much light entering the eye due to a damaged cornea (corneal abrasion), retinal damage, or pupil(s) unable to normally constrict (seen in cases of damage to the oculomotor nerve). This is also seen in albinism (a lack of pigment in the iris), where the irises can't completely block light from entering the eye.

Patients with photophobia will avoid direct light, and may seek the shelter of a dark room or wear sunglasses.

Please do not panic, but go to A&E or the ER if you think you or a child is unwell, and you cannot get an appointment in surgery or speak to a doctor.

If this symptom has a sudden onset, and the associated symptoms are red, please do not waste time asking for a nurse triage service or expecting doctors to visit you at home. Go to hospital and consult an eye specialist to help get a diagnosis and the right treatment.

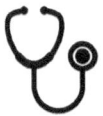 POISONING

If you are exposed to a substance that can damage your health or endanger your life, you must go to hospital.

In 2013–14, almost 150,000 people were admitted to hospital with poisoning in England.

Children under five have the highest risk of accidental poisoning. In one in four reported cases the person involved intentionally poisoned him or herself.

Symptoms depend on the type of poison and the amount taken in. If you are vomiting, have stomach pains, are confused, drowsy, and feel like fainting after an exposure to a harmful substance, you must go to hospital.

If a child suddenly develops these symptoms, and they are in the vicinity of some harmful substance (listed below), they may have been poisoned, particularly if they are drowsy and confused.

If you suspect that someone has taken an overdose or has been poisoned, don't try to treat them yourself. Go to hospital, or call 111.

If they are showing signs of being seriously ill, such as vomiting, loss of consciousness, drowsiness, or seizures (fits), call 999 to request an ambulance.

Poisons can be swallowed, absorbed through the skin, inhaled, splashed into the eyes, or injected.

A medication overdose is the most common form of poisoning in the UK. This can include over-the-counter medications, such as paracetamol, antidepressants, and hypnotics, or pesticides.

Other potential poisons include:

Dishwasher liquid, scouring soap, window cleaner, medicines, oven cleaner, vitamins, furniture polish, ammonia, washing powder, bleach, dyes, rat poison, ant poison, weed killer, pesticides,

petrol, car wash, anti–freeze, cosmetics, shampoo, nail polish, perfume, some types of plants and fungi, carbon monoxide (smoke), and recreational drugs. You can also be poisoned by poorly prepared or cooked food, food that has gone mouldy or been contaminated with bacteria from raw meat, and alcohol, if an excessive amount is consumed over a short period of time.

Snakes, and insects such as wasps and bees, aren't poisonous, but their bites or stings can contain venom (toxin).

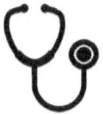 **POLYUREA**

This is common in elderly patients with heart failure, who are often taking water tablets that make them pass more urine.

This is not a common problem but, can be associated with hormonal changes, salt and water abnormalities, infection, and kidney or heart problems.

If you are vomiting and/or have other symptoms that are red, you must go to a hospital and get the right treatment soon. Please treat this as an acute presentation of a serious illness that requires an emergency appointment.

Diabetes is one of the most common causes of this symptom, and it is often associated with excessive thirst.

If you are forcing yourself to drink excess water because someone told you to drink more water every day, then the problem is likely to be what we call psychogenic polyuria and polydipsia.

If you are not very ill, get a blood sugar test done in a local pharmacist. If the sugar levels are high, make an appointment and consult a nurse.

Please make sure that the doctor or nurse checks your blood pressure.

If you have other associated symptoms like vomiting, behavioral changes, weakness, loss of weight, pain when passing urine, or blood in your urine, please treat this as an emergency.

 **POOR HEARING**

The most common cause of poor hearing when not associated with fever is impacted wax.

If the symptom is associated with fever your ear must be examined using a PNEUMATIC OTOSCOPE.

Some doctors and nurses assume that red ears are associated with infection, and prescribe antibiotics. But the eardrum can be red if the body temperature increases, after sneezing, or if a child has been crying for some time. We must stop this habit of abusing antibiotics.

Please make sure your ears are examined properly using a pneumatic otoscope and/or tuning fork (Webber and Renni test).

Please note that children with poor hearing have delayed speech. If your child is not speaking well, please consult an ENT specialist or speak to a Health visitor, and get a hearing test.

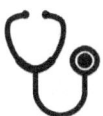 ## POST-MENOPAUSAL BLEEDING,

Please speak to a nurse or a doctor. If the bleeding is profuse, please treat this as an emergency and go to hospital. If the bleeding is on and off and small, consult your doctor or go to family planning clinic

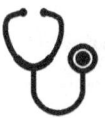 ## PREMATURE EJACULATION

Premature ejaculation is a common problem, associated with erectile dysfunction (ED) or impotence. It is a sexual dysfunction, A penile erection occurs when the blood enters the cavernous (sponge-like bodies) tissue within the penis. This process is initiated as a result of sexual arousal, when signals are transmitted from the brain via the nerves.

Diseases or disorders of the cardiovascular, or metabolic systems, and hormonal or neurological abnormalities can produce ED.

Drugs and psychological problems are more important than physiological problems in this case. ED can result in relationship difficulties and damage to the masculine self-image.

Besides treating the underlying causes such as potassium deficiency, or arsenic contamination of drinking water, the first-line treatments of erectile dysfunction consist of a trial of drugs like sildenafil (Viagra), which helps establish the cause.

Approximately 40% of males suffer from erectile dysfunction or impotence, at least occasionally.

Please consult your doctors, and if you married or having relationship issues, please contact the NGO, Relate and get help.

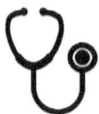 **PREGNANCY**

Are you pregnant? You won't notice any symptoms until about the time you've missed a period – or a week or two later.

If you're not monitoring your menstrual cycle, or if it varies from one month to the next, you may not be sure when to expect your period. But if you start to experience some of the symptoms listed below, please get a home pregnancy test or ask a chemist to perform a pregnancy test.

Tender, swollen breasts. This is one of the early signs of pregnancy – sensitive, sore breasts caused by increasing levels of hormones.

Feeling tired, exhaustion and fatigue. Rapidly increasing levels of the hormone progesterone can make you feel sleepy and look as if you are daydreaming.

Some women have a small amount of vaginal bleeding around 11 or 12 days after conception. This may be close to the time that you might notice a missed period. The fertilized egg burrowing into the blood-rich lining of your uterus may cause this bleeding.

Nausea or vomiting and early morning sickness is common. This can occur a month after conception, but some women do start vomiting a bit earlier. Some women vomit all day and night.

Increased sensitivity to odors, and potentially feeling nauseous. You may feel repelled by the smell of a bologna sandwich or cup of coffee, causing such aromas to trigger your gag reflex. This may be due to rapidly increasing amounts of oestrogen in your system. Certain foods may become suddenly completely repulsive to you.

Hormonal changes in early pregnancy may leave you feeling bloated, in a similar way to the feeling some women have just before their period arrives. Clothes may feel tighter than usual at the waistline, even early on, when your uterus is still quite small.

Increased urination, and hurrying to the bathroom all the time. During pregnancy the amount of blood and other fluids in your body increases, which leads to extra fluid being processed by your kidneys and ending up in your bladder.

Body metabolic rate and temperature stays high. If you've been charting your basal body temperature and you see that your temperature has stayed elevated for 18 days in a row, you're probably pregnant. A missed period is the first sign, if you're usually pretty regular and your period doesn't arrive on time. A pregnancy test confirms the diagnosis. But if you're not regular or you're not keeping track of your cycle, nausea and breast tenderness are the signs to watch out for.

Please get a home pregnancy test if you had unprotected sex and are missing periods, even if you are using alternative contraception.

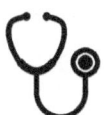 **RAPID WEIGHT GAIN,**

Rapid weight gain is often associated with the medical condition hypothyroidism (an underactive thyroid). In this case, the thyroid gland is not producing enough thyroid hormones, which are essential to regulating the body's metabolism. This can occur at any age and in either sex, though it is most common in older women. The body's metabolism slows down, which can lead to rapid weight gain. This condition is usually treated with daily hormone-replacement tablets, called levothyroxine.

Diabetic patients can rapidly gain weight due to the side effects of insulin. Patients on insulin eat more than they need to, in order to prevent low blood sugar. Excessive snacking to prevent a hypoglycemic attack contributes towards an excessive calorie intake and overall weight gain.

Elderly people begin to lose modest amounts of muscle because they are less active, potentially leading to weight gain.

Steroids are used to treat a variety of conditions, including asthma and arthritis. Steroids can increase appetite in some people, leading to weight gain.

Cushing's syndrome affects around one in 50,000 people, and is caused by high levels of the hormone cortisol. This can develop as a side effect of long-term steroid treatment (iatrogenic Cushing's syndrome), or as the result of a tumor (endogenous Cushing's syndrome). Weight gain is a common symptom, particularly on the chest, face and stomach. It occurs because the hormone cortisol causes fat to be redistributed to these areas.

People respond differently to stress, anxiety, and depression. Some people lose weight, while others gain weight.

People who sleep less than seven hours a day/night may be more likely to be overweight than those who get nine hours of sleep or more.

Fluid retention causes parts of the body to become swollen. Premenstrual swelling can occur in one particular part of the body, such as the ankles, or can be more general. More severe fluid retention can also cause breathlessness.

Polycystic ovaries are a common condition that affects how a woman's ovaries work. Symptoms can include irregular periods, trouble getting pregnant, excess hair, and weight gain.

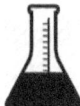
RASH COMES AND GOES

This is probably the most common cause of itchy skin. This symptom may be associated with puffiness and redness around the eyes and lips if the cause is a generalized allergic reaction.

Along with the itchiness, there will most probably be problems with breathing, the throat and nose, and possibly even a headache.

If the itchy rash is experienced mostly in the spring, or the time that allergies often affect sufferers, it is probably an allergic reaction. The rash can be local if you touched some plant or weeds.

If you have been exposed to something that you are allergic to, the body will release histamine that will spread all over body via the blood.

This rash will blanch (fade) with pressure, but can often be frightening to see.

The treatment is antihistamines. These can be bought in the chemist. If breathlessness and/or swollen lips occur, you must rush to the hospital A&E or ER.

Please consult a doctor soon to get tests and identify what you are allergic to.

Some doctors do not perform the tests, and simply making a note of substances you are allergic to can be more than enough. Eczema, scabies, and liver disease also produce a generalized itchy rash.

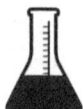 ## RASH ITCHY

The most common cause of an itchy rash is an allergic reaction. If this symptom is accompanied by puffiness and redness around the eyes, swollen lips, and/or breathlessness, you must rush to the hospital A&E or ER.

Please consult a doctor soon to get tests and identify what you are allergic to.

If the itchy eyes are experienced mostly in the spring, the time that allergies often affect sufferers, or if you know that you have been exposed to something that you are allergic to, then it is pretty obvious what is causing the itching.

The rash will blanch (fade) with pressure but can often be frightening to see.

The treatment is antihistamines. These can be bought in the chemist. Please consult a doctor soon to get tests and identify what you are allergic to.

Some doctors do not perform the tests, and simply making a note of substances you are allergic to can be more than enough. Eczema, scabies, and liver disease also produce a generalized itchy rash.

If you are pregnant and experience itching, please let your obstetrician or doctor know about this.

Itching at night is often due to bed bugs, scabies or something in the bedroom that you are allergic to.

 ## RASH ITCHY AFTER HOT BATH

You feel comfortable taking a hot bath to ease the itch, but the rash is reddish and very itchy after a hot bath. Itching is often worst in the night.

Often doctors and nurses have made the mistake of this symptom as eczema and have been using steroid cream.

The itch is occurring because the body is producing chemicals to fight invading allergens. Steroids suppress this immune response and so infestations like scabies will spread all over the body.

This is a typical case of a rash appearing on your skin when you sleep in bed.

The cause is usually bed bugs and/or scabies. Scabies produce borrows in the skin and hide.

You will see the burrows, but scabies are very tiny and can only be seen with a microscope. Some doctors request skin scraping microscopy, but this is not mandatory.

An experienced doctor will diagnose this cause, and often treat it using creams and shampoos. The rash is common in the axilla and groin areas.

Scabies can be transferred during sexual contact, so you must be careful when you go to a massage parlour or to brothels.

Secondary bacterial infection is common. If this develops, you must get treatment to clear the bacterial infection first and then start antifungal treatment.

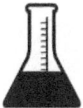 ## RASH LOOKS LIKE CHICKEN POX

Chicken pox spots are typically round, with slight turbid fluid inside. If other children in the area have had chicken pox, the chances of your child or you getting chicken pox are high.

You can find images of the rash published on the Internet. Please speak to a chemist and get treatment.

Visiting the doctor's surgery and/or A&E is not a good idea, because your child or you may catch another infection.

You may also infect other patients who are in the waiting area. If you are worried, speak to your doctors, or call 111.

Chicken pox lesions are often present in the mouth and vagina. Treatment is only symptomatic.

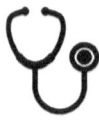

RASH DOES NOT DISAPPEAR WITH PRESSURE

This rash is usually purple, does not disappear with pressure or after you place a glass against it.

The rash is not painful, but spreads all over the body very rapidly.

This non-blanching rash is serious, and you must rush to hospital.

Please call emergency services and inform them that you may have an infectious disease, so they must come prepared with protective uniforms.

If the rash blanches (fades) with pressure, then it is probably the result of an allergic reaction (see elsewhere). Treatment is antihistamines. These can be bought in the chemist. If breathlessness and/or swollen lips occur, you must rush to the hospital A&E or ER.

The diagnosis of this symptom requires proper clinical examination, isolation and investigation.

Doctors will only treat this symptom after ruling out serious illnesses, so you must consult a doctor.

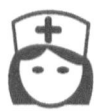

RED COLORED RASH

If the rash is hot, this is likely to be infection.

Impetigo secretes turbid fluid and crusts on the skin.

A red rash which is painful may be an abscess or erythematous rash, associated with infections.

Please get a nurse to take a look, or consult a dermatologist.

Please do not borrow others' cream or ointments.

You must not use steroids or antibiotics without knowing what organism or allergy caused the rash.

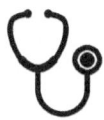

RED OR PURPLE RASH

This rash is usually purple, does not disappear with pressure or after you place a glass against it.

The rash is not painful, but spreads all over the body very rapidly.

This non-blanching rash is serious, and you must rush to hospital.

Please call emergency services and inform them that you may have an infectious disease, so they must come prepared with protective uniforms.

If the rash blanches (fades) with pressure, then it is probably the result of an allergic reaction (see elsewhere). Treatment is antihistamines. These can be bought in the chemist. If breathlessness and/or swollen lips occur, you must rush to the hospital A&E or ER.

The diagnosis of this symptom requires proper clinical examination, isolation and investigation.

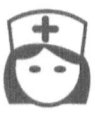

RED RASH

If the rash is red and hot, this is likely to be an infection.

Impetigo secretes turbid fluid and crusts on the skin.

A red rash which is painful may be an abscess or erythematous rash, associated with infections.

Please get a nurse to take a look, or consult a dermatologist.

Please do not borrow creams or treatment used by others.

You must not use steroids or antibiotics without knowing what organism or allergy caused the rash.

Reddish areas around lacerations, open wounds, or suture sites can have a bluish discoloration around the wound when the wound is fresh.

An infection will also cause the edges to be blue, but you will have other associated symptoms.

If pus or a watery discharge is seen, the wound may have an infection.

Bacteria that infect wounds are resistant to treatment.

Taking antibiotics orally, using antibiotic creams, ointments, or alcohol washes can cause more harm than good.

Please consult a doctor.

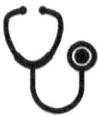 **REDUCED VISION**

This is a common symptom associated with vertigo, head injuries, alcohol intoxication, drugs, and infections.

There are numerous causes, and you will need to be reviewed by an ophthalmologist. Please go to a walk-in-eye clinic, or go to hospital.

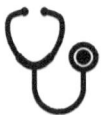 **RETURNED FROM HOLIDAY**

Common symptoms of illness can occur after a holiday. The illness is likely to be different depending on what you were exposed to, so please choose your symptoms.

Symptoms like diarrhoea, vomiting, high fever, rash, headache and stool containing blood and mucus, are all worth noting. Please speak to your doctor first before you rush to hospital.

Infections like typhoid, malaria, cholera, and amoebic dysentery are common in the tropics.

Emerging infections like Ebola, MERS, SARS, resistant TB, Typhoid, and even sexually transmitted diseases are spreading all over the world, and so you must speak to a doctor if you feel unwell after travelling abroad.

You may have vague symptoms like a rash that does not look serious. Please speak to a doctor, as you may be referred to a tropical disease specialist for advice and treatment.

Doctors will perform tests, scans, and chest X-Rays, or refer you to specialist care.

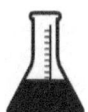 **RING WORM**

Ringworm (Tinea) can affect many parts of the body, particularly the groin and scalp.

It is most noticeable on bare skin, where it is referred to as ringworm due to its characteristic appearance as a circular patch of red, itchy skin, which gradually increases in size.

There may also be red, itchy areas around the bases of hair shafts.

With scratching, these areas can bleed and become crusted with blood. This symptom is caused by a fungus, not a worm.

Prevention: Keep the area well ventilated and dry. Use a separate face cloth and towel. Do not use those of other people. Ringworm is infectious.

Complications: a bacterial infection from scratching is common.

Self-care: keep the area well ventilated and dry. Use a cream or special shampoo as recommended by your pharmacist.

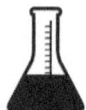 ## RUNNY NOSE

This is a very common symptom that has often been managed poorly. People assume that a runny nose is a sign of a "Cold" or "FLU," which is caused by a virus and will get better soon.

A watery secretion dripping from the nose is a normal bodily response to trap dust, allergens and/or micro-organisms, and prevent them entering the lungs.

The medical term used to describe this symptom is "Rhinitis."

Managing this symptom is easy, but problems occur because people do not follow instructions properly. The way to help reduce secretions is by blocking allergens from touching the nasal mucosa.

This treatment is available in the local chemist. Please try to self-treat this symptom before consulting a doctor.

Doctors who understand patho-physiology will offer a nasal spray first, but others may prescribe antibiotics.

A nasal spray containing mild steroids can block the inflammatory process that produces watery secretions in the nose. This will stop the nose from being runny or blocked. Otrivine Adult Metered Dose 0.1% xylometazoline hydrochloride Nasal Spray delivers a precise dose of medicated spray to the inside of the nose, which will block the production of secretions. It provides up to 10 hours of relief in as little as 2 minutes. It contains the active ingredient xylometazoline hydrochloride that helps to open up and clear the nasal passages by reducing nasal mucus and returning swollen blood vessels to their normal size.

Please note that this drug will make the symptom worse if used regularly for more than 3–5 days.

If the problem is chronic, please do not assume you have the common cold.

Please read all about "Rhinitis" and get the correct treatment.

Please note that there is no drug that cures this condition, only those which offer symptomatic treatment – your symptom will be relieved only when you are using the nasal spray.

If the symptom persists for a long time, the chances of your getting a bacterial infection are high, and so you may need antibiotics. If you do, the treatment must be continued for six weeks and then stopped.

Please do not stop treatment after the symptom resolves, because the drug only works for 12–24 hours, and then the symptom will return.

 ## SCABIES

Although intensely itchy, scabies is rarely a serious condition.

Scabies is caused by a mite, which burrows just under the skin, often between the fingers, on wrists, elbows and the genital areas causing a red rash. It can only come from contact with infected people. Red lines, which follow the burrows of the mite as it travels into the skin, soon merge with the inevitable scratching. It is usually worse at night when the mite is most active.

Bacterial infections from excessive scratching can make the situation worse.

Please do not use steroid cream, because this will help spread scabies, and a bacterial infection will occur.

Ointments are available from your pharmacist. All of the body will need to be covered with the ointment for 24 hours, and all clothing and bedding should be washed thoroughly.

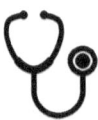 ## SEPTICEMIA

Septicaemia occurs when bacteria or viruses enter the blood. Its common name is Blood Poisoning. This is actually a complication of infection. The duty of a doctor is to identify the infection, and treat it with the right antibiotic, in order to prevent septicaemia.

39,000 patients die in the UK every year because primary care doctors and nurses have failed to identify and/or treat common infections early.

Meningitis is associated with septicaemia. This occurs when bacteria from the blood enters the brain, producing an inflammation of the brain lining which can be fatal. Unfortunately, the symptoms can be easily mistaken for flu or a bad cold.

Worse still, it is more difficult to be certain with babies and young children. If you are not sure, you must call 111.

Hib immunization has reduced the number of people suffering from some types of meningitis or septicaemia.

Symptoms in babies under 2 years old: the babies can be difficult to wake, their cry may be high pitched and different from normal, they may vomit repeatedly, and not just after feeds, may refuse feeds, either from the bottle, the breast, or by spoon. Their skin may appear pale or blotchy, possibly with a red/purple rash, which does not fade when you press a tumbler glass or a finger against the rash.

The soft spot on top of your baby's head (the fontanels) may be tight or bulging.

The baby may seem irritable and dislike being handled.

The baby's body may be floppy, or else stiff with jerky movements. Remember that a fever may not be present in the early stages.

Older children may have slightly different symptoms:

A constant generalized headache, a high temperature, although their hands and feet may be cold, vomiting, drowsiness, confusion, and sensitivity to bright lights, daylight, or even the TV.

Neck stiffness – moving their chin to their chest will be very painful at the back of the neck.

A rash of red or purple spots or bruises, which does not fade when you press a tumbler glass or a finger against the rash. The rash may not be present in the early stages.

Other, rarer symptoms: Joint or muscle pain, rapid breathing, stomach pain, sometimes with diarrhoea.

Symptoms can appear in any order and not everyone gets all of the symptoms.

There are different types of bacteria and viruses that can produce meningitis and/or septicaemia.

A vaccination programme has now started for meningitis C for children and young people up to 17 years of age. Some forms of meningitis do not, as yet, have a vaccination, so the disease can still occur.

Note that people who have been in contact with someone who has had meningitis should contact a close relative of the patient to find out any instructions (from the hospital or the Director of Public Health) that they may have been given regarding antibiotics. Otherwise your doctor will be able to give you appropriate advice. Only those who have been in very close contact with the infected person are given antibiotics and vaccinations in response.

 ## SHINGLES

This rash is confined to one side of the body, and is restricted to one area because the rash is present in the dermatome (the area supplied by the nerve).

This is the same virus which causes chicken pox.

Shingles does not occur if you did not have chicken pox as a child, but children and adults not immune to chickenpox can get infected with chickenpox if they come in contact with a patient suffering from shingles.

If the rash is noticed in young adults, please consult your GP to get a blood check.

Shingles occurs when the body's immunity is low, and so you may need various tests. It is particularly nasty if the immune system is not working properly, such as during another illness, or while receiving treatment for cancer. Please consult a doctor.

It is rare to develop shingles more than once.

The initial symptom is often a tingling itchy feeling, preceding a painful rash only found on one side of the body. This can develop over the next few hours or days into a painful set of blisters.

The rash usually follows a narrow strip of skin; common sites include the chest wall, face, and upper legs.

A general flu-like illness often accompanies the rash, which may persist after the rash has gone.

If you have never had chicken pox you are very unlikely to develop shingles, which is caused by the same virus.

Prevention is difficult; most people will develop this infection without realizing where it came from.

Although sometimes very painful, shingles is rarely serious. People who are suffering from any condition which lowers their resistance to infection, or on medications that have a similar effect, can be quite ill. If the infection spreads onto the tip of the nose, it may affect the eye, and immediate attention from your doctor is recommended should this happen.

Once the tingling sensation begins, it is wise to start an antiviral medicine like acyclovir (e.g., Zovirax). Although it is possible to treat the infection with acyclovir (e.g., Zovirax), it is important to start treatment as soon as possible once the itchiness starts. Once the rash is well developed, acyclovir is of no great value.

If the rash is painful, please wrap cling film around it. This will help to ease the pain and discomfort.

Simple painkillers such as aspirin and paracetamol will help.

Keep the rash area uncovered as much as possible.

Try not to scratch the rash.

Use calamine lotion to ease the itchiness.

Cooling the area with a bag of ice can reduce the pain which follows the disappearance of the rash.

See your doctor, especially if:

- The blisters occur near your eye, or on the tip of your nose.
- Pain is not healed after ten days.
- This symptom is associated with high temperature.
- You have some other serious illness.
- Your eyes are sore and red.

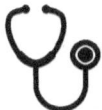 ## SKIN IS YELLOW

Having a yellow tinge to the skin, or the whites of the eyes is often a sign that you have a mild attack of jaundice.

If the whites of your eyes are yellow, then it is quite likely that your skin will be too. Jaundice produces chemicals which accumulate in oily skin and the eyes.

Jaundice is quite common in new-borns, but it can affect people at any age, and be variable in its intensity. If an affected baby is not feeding well, and is drowsy and lethargic, please consult a doctor because the baby may develop long-term problems. Please make sure the baby is feeding well, because low sugar will allow jaundice to enter the brain resulting in kernicterus.

Jaundice is what happens when bilirubin builds up in our body tissue and in the blood.

The most common causes for this build-up of bilirubin are a liver condition, such as hepatitis, or the presence of gallstones.

If you have a yellowing of the whites of the eyes as well as a tinge of yellow to your skin, also look at the mucous membranes of the nose and mouth, which may also have taken on a yellow hue. This is cirrhosis of the liver.

When you go to the toilet, you might notice that the urine you pass is darker in color, and that your stools are lighter (whitish) in color.

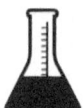 ## SNEEZING EXCESSIVE

Most of us will sneeze at one time or another. This is a reflex to prevent dust, allergens, or smoke damaging the lungs.

Although this is not usually very serious, it can be very irritating if the symptoms continue.

This symptom will always be associated with other symptoms.

An allergic reaction is probably the most common cause of excessive sneezing, and is often associated with itchiness in the eyes and/or puffiness and redness around the eyes.

Along with the itchiness, there will probably be problems with the throat and the nose, and possibly even the head as well.

If the sneezing is experienced mostly in the spring, the time that allergies most often affect sufferers, or if you know that you have been exposed to something that you are allergic to, then it will be pretty obvious what is causing the itching.

Colds and sinus infections can make you sneeze. Since the symptoms are very similar to an allergy, it is important to know which one you are actually suffering from.

If you are not sure what you have, and this symptom is associated with itchy eyes, a cough and a sore throat, please consult a chemist.

Hay fever is the most common cause of this and the drugs that will help reduce symptoms are available in pharmacies and need no prescription.

Conjunctivitis and other eye infections in babies and children may be associated with sneezing. The secretions from the eye are drained through the nose, so a blocked nose will often result in watery secretions dripping back into the throat. Babies may cough or sneeze as a result.

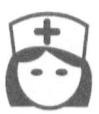 ## SOILING IN BED

This is a common problem, often seen in nursing homes, among the long-term mentally insane, and among elderly patients in hospital.

The majority of adults with this symptom have dementia, or have complicated illnesses that prevent them from moving from their bed. Arthritic, cardiac, or respiratory illnesses that prevent patients from walking too fast are also important factors.

This may or may not be associated with bed wetting.

If you are suffering from this problem, and are on benefits or welfare, please mention this to your doctor, as you are likely to get extra help to make your life comfortable.

Diarrhoea, constipation, and anal disorders are also associated with soiling.

Infections and infestation in children or the elderly are some common causes.

Please discuss this with a doctor, and get the right diagnosis and treatment.

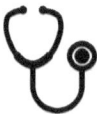

SQUINT

A sudden onset squint is associated with serious eye problems.

A squint in babies less than a week old must be referred to an ophthalmologist.

An ophthalmologist must see a child with constant squinting as early as possible.

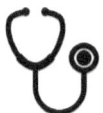

STOOLS BLACK OR TARRY

Blood entering the intestine will be digested, and the iron content of the red cells will stain stools black. Fresh bleeding seen in the stool is unlikely to be from the intestine, so is less worrying.

The diagnosis of this symptom requires proper clinical examination, and will require investigation. The bleeding is internal, so you will require a colonoscopy to identify the cause and stop the bleeding.

The common causes of this are gastritis, ulcers, using drugs like non-steroidal anti-inflammatories (e.g., brufen, aspirin, diclofenac), and polyps.

Doctors will only treat this symptom after ruling out all of these conditions, so please consult a DOCTOR.

Please do not panic, but go to A&E, and please do not wait to get an appointment. If possible, speak to a doctor.

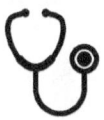 **STRUGGLING TO BREATHEE**

This is what we call "Central Cyanosis" indicating that blood is not getting enough oxygen and so is turning blue.

Please do not waste time, but call an ambulance and go to hospital now.

The doctors will examine the patient to differentiate between heart, lungs, and circulation problems.

If this is a symptom in a child, please do not ignore it, but call an ambulance, and go to hospital.

If the child struggles to breathe when playing or eating, the most likely cause is a foreign body aspiration, which must be managed in hospitals as an emergency.

You will also notice that the symptoms associated with this are likely to be red.

Doctors will perform examinations, investigations, blood tests, scans, and may request a bronchoscopy.

Please do not try to open the mouth, because this will cause the foreign body to be sucked further in, and make the obstruction of the airway worse.

 SWELLING AROUND JAW

Local injury and mumps are some of the common conditions that can cause swelling around the jaw.

Mumps:

The incubation period of mumps is 12–28 days. The patient is infectious from 3 days prior to the swelling until 7 days after it resolves.

This illness is characterized by swelling or pain in the parotid glands and sub-mandibular area (in front of the ears and neck), a dry mouth, worse pain on swallowing or chewing, a fever (high to very high), malaise, headache, drowsiness, vomiting, abdominal (tummy) pain, and photophobia: cannot stand bright light. This may also be associated with testicular pain.

This was once a common disease in children, which became very rare following the introduction of the mumps vaccination. Unfortunately, this disease is likely to return, as viruses and bacteria are becoming resistant to treatment and learning to overcome immunity.

There may be mild prodromal symptoms prior to the swelling of the salivary glands. Parotid glands (below the ears) are nearly always affected.

Women must get a pregnancy test, as this infection can damage the foetus.

Most cases are without serious consequence, but complications include orchitis, pancreatitis, viral meningitis, and the risk of miscarriage between 12 and 16 weeks' gestation.

Paracetamol or ibuprofen help reduce the pain and fever, and you should maintain a high fluid intake.

Avoid acidic fruit juices, because it may increase the pain and should be avoided.

Go to hospital if:

There is abdominal pain in the left side radiating to back: Pancreatitis caused by infected pancreases.

Testicular pain is present: Orchitis is rare before puberty, usually unilateral and rarely, if ever, causes infertility.

Oophoritis – infected ovaries, if you are pregnant, give this special attention.

SWELLING AROUND WOUND

This is a common problem, because inflammation is a process that causes blood circulation to an area to increase.

The body is trying to fight off infection.

If this symptom is associated with other red symptoms, please consult a doctor, or go to hospital.

SWELLING IN THE NECK

The most common cause of this condition is a thyroid problem.

Please consult a doctor to get the diagnosis confirmed by a Thyroid Function Test (TSH, T3 and T4).

This is a very common condition in teenagers, but is often not recognized or diagnosed. The reason teenagers do not report this is because they tend to eat a lot but do not gain weight.

Doctors are said to abuse thyroxin to help them lose weight.

People with thyroid problems can suffer from heavy periods, and they are often anxious and have palpitations.

This issue produces a high metabolic rate, and so the patient burns too many calories.

This can lead to long-term psychological problems like anxiety attacks and acute psychosis. It can also affect the heart, and may lead to an acute "thyrotoxicosis crisis" that can be difficult to manage.

Please consult a doctor and make sure you get treatment.

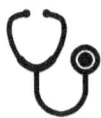 **SWOLLEN LEGS**

Swollen legs are often associated with a heart problem. You must consult a doctor as soon as possible.

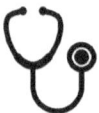 **SWOLLEN TESTES**

The common term used by doctors for swollen testes is hydrocele. This is a very common symptom, often seen in babies and children.

The important factor that determines the difference between the various issues that can cause this is the onset and duration of the symptom.

If you notice that the symptom has existed for some time, but it is not associated with pain or any other symptoms, this is unlikely to be an emergency problem. You will need a correct diagnosis and treatment, however.

If the symptom has existed for some time, but you have an acute onset of pain, then the chances of strangulated hernias, testicular torsion, or infections like orchitis are high, so you must consult a doctor as an emergency.

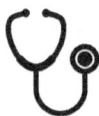
SWOLLEN TUMMY

When fluid slowly accumulates between the lining of the abdomen wall and the organs, this is known as ascites.

Please note that the distension occurs in periods of short duration. Arms, waist and legs may not be soft, but are often thin.

This is not very common, but is often missed because people assume they are getting obese.

Ascites usually occurs when the liver stops working properly, or the blood pressure in the liver and pancreas increases (portal hypertension). Fluid fills the space between the lining of the abdomen and the organs.

Liver scarring is a common cause of ascites. Scars will increase pressure inside the liver's blood vessels, forcing fluid into the abdominal cavity, and causing ascites.

Liver damage from sources such as cirrhosis, hepatitis B or C infection, alcohol abuse, and heart or kidney failure are the common causes of ascites.

Other conditions that may increase your risk of ascites include: ovarian, pancreatic, liver, or endometrial cancer, pancreatitis, and tuberculosis.

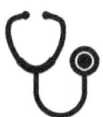
SWALLOWING DIFFICULTY

The most common cause of this symptom is infection. The key is to differentiate between bacterial and viral infections. The diagnosis of this symptom requires proper clinical examination, and may require investigation. Doctors will only treat this symptom after ruling out serious illnesses so please consult a DOCTOR, and not a nurse in the UK. Please do not panic, but go to A&E if you cannot get an appointment, or you cannot speak to or consult a doctor.

TALKING FUNNY

This is a common symptom that is associated with very high fever. Doctors use the word "delirious" to refer to this symptom. Patients who have dementia, or other long-term illness, who start talking funny or have behavioral problems must be investigated to rule out infection. The most common cause is a urinary infection. This problem is also associated with viral infections, but doctors find it hard to be 100% certain that this is a viral infection. The diagnosis of this symptom requires proper clinical examination, and may require investigation. Doctors will only treat this symptom after ruling out serious illnesses so please consult a DOCTOR. Please do not panic, but go to A&E or the ER if you cannot get an appointment, or you cannot speak to or consult a doctor.

THROAT HAS WHITE SPOTS

White spots on the tonsils, and a recurrent sore throat is often caused by the BE virus. The common term used for this is glandular fever. There are a few painless, swollen lymph nodes on the neck. Some bacteria like mycoplasma and streptococcus can produce whitish spots on the tonsils. You need to treat this with large doses of antibiotics. Please note that a serious widespread rash will occur if you prescribe amoxicillin/penicillin. Glandular fever must first be ruled out. A simple blood test can confirm the diagnosis. It is important to keep doing some activity, and to make sure you stay positive and get better. There is no antibiotic to cure glandular fever, because the infection is viral.

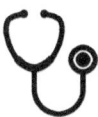

THROAT LUMP

The diagnosis of this symptom requires proper clinical examination, and investigation. This is not common, because a lump in the throat is caused by an infection. The common term used is "quincy." The treatment of this condition is surgical, so it must be treated by specialists in the hospital. Doctors will only treat this symptom after ruling out serious illnesses, so you must consult a doctor or go to A&E or the ER.

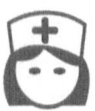

THRUSH IN MOUTH

This is a common symptom caused by a fungus – candida – in babies, and also in people who are immunosuppressed (on steroids or cancer treatment, or have an immunodeficiency). This is a simple problem, but often managed poorly by doctors and nurses because they do not make clear how to treat it. Babies will often cry and have difficulty feeding. This is not a common symptom in adults; please consult doctors if you have this symptom. You will be investigated, and properly treated with the right drug if necessary. Delays in diagnosis can result in complications, which can result in long-term illness. Please note that you must give oral antifungal gel after feeding and also use a nappy antifungal cream every time you change the nappy. If you are using ever-dry nappies, please keep the affected area open and exposed to air. The treatment must be given for at least 5 days.

Make sure you get a new set of teats or dummies, and heat wash if you are using reusable nappies. A relapse, or recurrent nappy rash or oral thrush occurs because you have not fully cleared the infection.

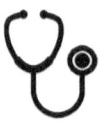 ## TINGLING SENSATION

This is a symptom associated with the superficial nerves, and you must consult a doctor about it, preferably a neurologist.

A tingling sensation in the finger tips and/or toes is associated with anxiety or panic attacks.

Please do not self-diagnose this, or delay in getting the correct diagnosis and treatment.

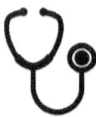 ## TINNITUS

Tinnitus is a common problem, said to affect about 1 in 5 people. It may be caused by an underlying condition, such as age related hearing loss, an ear injury, or a circulatory system disorder.

This is not a sign of a serious illness, but it can worsen with age.

Tinnitus is treated by dealing with the underlying cause, or by taking drugs to reduce or mask the noise, making tinnitus less noticeable.

Tinnitus involves the annoying sensation of hearing sounds that may be described as a ringing, buzzing, roaring, clicking or hissing, that may be present all the time, or may come and go.

There are two kinds of tinnitus: subjective tinnitus, and objective tinnitus.

Tinnitus may be associated with hearing loss or dizziness.

In many cases, an exact cause is never found.

A common cause of tinnitus is inner-ear cell damage.

Other causes of tinnitus include other ear problems, age related hearing loss, exposure to loud sound, impacted wax, or a blocked ear, ear bone changes (otosclerosis), TMJ disorders, head or neck injuries, acoustic neuroma, drugs, chronic health conditions, and injuries or conditions that affect the nerves in your ear or the hearing center in your brain.

Tinnitus can also be an early indicator of Meniere's disease, an inner-ear disorder that may be caused by abnormal inner-ear fluid pressure.

Please consult a doctor if the tinnitus persists or is a sudden onset.

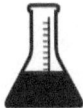 **TRAVEL SICKNESS**

This is also known as travel sickness, motion sickness, seasickness, carsickness, or airsickness. It is a combination of dizziness, nausea, and vomiting that can occur when you travel.

You may also look pale, feel cold, experience an increase in saliva production, have tummy rumbles, and/or start vomiting.

Rare associated symptoms are rapid, shallow breathing, feeling drowsy, headaches, and feeling very tired.

These symptoms will start to improve as your body adapts to the conditions causing the problem. If you have motion sickness on a cruise ship, the symptoms will get better after a couple of days.

Anyone can get motion sickness, but some are more vulnerable than others. Women often experience motion sickness, particularly during menstruation (periods), or pregnancy. People with a history of recurrent headaches or migraines are more likely to suffer.

Travel sickness is more common in children aged 3 to 12, but will generally resolve as they get older.

It's only necessary to seek medical advice about motion sickness if your symptoms continue after you stop travelling. Your GP will then be able to rule out other possible causes of your symptoms, such as a viral infection of your inner-ear (labyrinthitis).

This symptom occurs when there is a conflict between what your eyes see, and what your inner ears, which help with balance, sense.

Your brain holds details about where you are, and how you are moving. It constantly updates this with information from your eyes and vestibular system.

The vestibular system is a network of nerves, channels, and fluids in your inner-ear, which give your brain a sense of motion and balance.

If there is a mismatch of information between these two systems, your brain can't update your current status, and the resulting confusion will lead to the symptoms of motion sickness, such as nausea and vomiting.

There is also an association between motion sickness and a type of migraine where dizziness, rather than the headache, dominates. This is known as a vestibular migraine. If you experience dizzy spells, and have a history of motion sickness, you may be diagnosed as having vestibular migraines.

Management: Mild symptoms improve if you fix your eyes on the horizon or a distant object, or confuse the brain by listening to music.

Stay still and do not read or play games.

Choose a cabin or seat in the middle of a boat or plane, because this is where you'll experience the least movement. Use a pillow or headrest to help keep your head still.

Closing your eyes may help relieve symptoms.

Fresh air – open windows in the car, or move to the top deck of a ship to avoid getting too hot and to get a good supply of fresh air.

Relax by listening to music while focusing on your breathing. Try counting backwards from 100- 99, 98, 97....

Avoid getting anxious, and stay calm. You're more likely to get motion sickness if you worry about it.

Avoid eating a large meal or drinking alcohol before travelling. You should keep well hydrated throughout your journey by drinking water.

Take medication for motion sickness before your journey to prevent symptoms from developing.

Hyoscine (scopolamine) is widely used to treat motion sickness. It's thought to work by blocking some of the nerve signals sent from the vestibular system. This drug is available over the counter from pharmacists. You must take the drug before travelling.

If you're going on a long journey by road, sea, or air; try applying hyoscine patches to your skin every three days.

Please read the instructions provided in the box, and discuss possible side effects with the chemist.

Antihistamines used to treat allergies are safe and help to control nausea and vomiting. They are less effective at treating motion sickness than hyoscine, but may cause fewer side effects.

Medication must be taken one or two hours before your journey.

If it is a long journey, you may need to take a dose every eight hours.

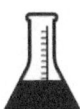 ## TUMMY BLOATING

This may be a sign of IBS. If so, diagnosis will be based on the exclusion of any other conditions. There is no definitive test for IBS, which affects three times as many women as men. Symptoms can start at any age, but appear predominantly in people between 15 and 40 years old. Stress and lifestyle factors are major considerations. The cause of IBS remains unknown, but it is rarely, if ever, fatal. Along with excessive wind, the symptoms of IBS are intermittent constipation, diarrhoea, and colicky tummy pain (abdominal pain). The cause of this illness is unknown, but it may be stress related or because your tummy is colonized with bad bacteria (common after taking antibiotics).

You should try a high-fibre diet containing wholegrain bread, rice, and pasta. Eating plenty of fresh fruit can produce a remarkable long-term improvement in symptoms. Dairy products are often the worst.

Try eliminating cheese, milk, chocolate, butter and cream from your diet for a few weeks to see if there is any improvement.

All red meat, not just beef, can often seriously upset your bowel if you are prone to IBS.

Use herbs known to alleviate the symptoms of IBS, e.g., peppermint. Stress can be a big factor.

Exercise increases bowel activity, thus reducing bloating and distension. Nicotine stimulates receptors in the bowel which can make your IBS much worse.

Small amounts of alcohol can actually help to stimulate gentle bowel function.

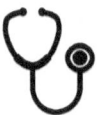 ## TUMMY PAIN

Please note that this is a common symptom, but must be examined by doctors to differentiate minor from serious illnesses.

Please speak to a doctor before taking any treatment, or go to hospital to consult a doctor as an emergency.

Please choose "Pain Abdomen" for more information.

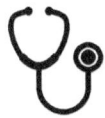 # UNABLE TO BREATH

The medical term used to describe this symptom is "Breathlessness."

This is a common complaint, but is a difficult symptom for a doctor to give advice on over the telephone, because you must be clinically examined, and may need a chest X-Ray, scan and other tests to confirm the diagnosis.

If the symptom is associated with other symptoms such as severe chest pain lasting more than 15 minutes, vomiting, and pain radiating to the jaw or arms – please call an ambulance and go to hospital.

Sudden onset breathlessness is not a common symptom, and must always be treated as a medical emergency.

Chest infections caused by bacteria often present with mild to moderate fever, followed by breathlessness and no cough. The proper name of chest infection is "pneumonia," and it must be treated as an emergency.

Oral antibiotics are not the right treatment, and you should not start a course of them. You will need intra-venous antibiotics given in large doses. Antibiotics given by mouth are poorly absorbed and so will only kill the good bacteria and provide an opportunity for resistant bacteria to grow.

Anxiety attacks, panic, and stress can also make some people complain of catching breath or air hunger, and often creates associated symptoms like palpitations (audible heart sounds), tachycardia (increased heart rate), and a tingling sensation in the fingers and/or toes.

If the symptom is acute and you feel dizzy, please call 999 and ask for an ambulance to take you to hospital. Please do not drive.

Asthma, chest infections, aspiration and acidosis are some of the common conditions that can cause breathlessness. These are illnesses that can only be managed in hospitals

This symptom is often associated with other red symptoms, but please treat this as an emergency and consult a doctor even if this happens to be the only red symptom. Please go to A&E or the ER.

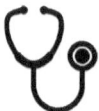

UNABLE TO SEE BRIGHT LIGHT

The diagnosis of this symptom requires proper clinical examination and may require investigations. This is a common symptom associated with meningitis, but there are other conditions like migraines and infections that can be associated with it. Doctors will only treat this symptom after ruling out serious illnesses, so you must consult a doctor.

This is typically a symptom of meningitis but can also occur in allergic conjunctivitis. It is difficult to differentiate these two so please go to hospital and do not wait to consult a GP.

Please do not panic, but go to A&E if you cannot get an appointment, or you cannot speak to or consult a doctor.

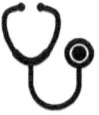

UNABLE TO SLEEP

Food, water, oxygen, and sleep are essential for humans and animals to live.

A lack of sleep makes you lethargic, unable to concentrate, have mood swings, and also develop other illnesses due to hormonal imbalance.

Some people require only four or five hours' sleep a night, whereas others need ten hours or more.

The amount of sleep required tends to lessen with age, and also with lower activity levels. A 'good night's sleep' is not the same for everyone. People who are burnt out often have sleep problems.

Almost everyone will have periods of insomnia at some stage. Extroverts are alert during the night and so work more at night. They often sleep once every two or three days for 12–18 hours. This is called catch-up sleep and rarely needs treatment.

REM (Rapid Eye Movement) sleep is important. This is the last stage of sleep. People who do not get REM often find it hard to relax, and may lack energy and feel they are depressed.

Early morning waking is a good indication that you may be depressed.

You need to answer the following questions:

What is your concern about the sleeping pattern?

When did this problem start, and what else was happening at that time?

Are you finding it difficult to get off to sleep?

Are you waking up often during the night?

Are you waking up in the early morning feeling tired?

What was your previous pattern like?

Do you take daytime naps?

Does your partner say that you snore and are restless?

What are your expectations of treatment?

Common causes are: Excessive caffeine, nicotine, alcohol, recreational drugs, and lifestyle factors – e.g., shift work.

A more complete list of potential causes is given below:

Physical: pain, itching, shortness of breath, nocturia, indigestion, tinnitus, discomfort, too warm, too cold, noise, room not dark enough.

Physiological: shift work, jet lag, and pregnancy.

Psychological: emotional upsets, worries, and bereavement.

Psychiatric: especially depression, or hypomania.

Pathological: sleep apnoea, restless leg syndrome.

Pharmacological: is the patient on any medication which might cause insomnia, e.g., corticosteroids, propranolol, pseudoephedrine or laxatives, or taking in excessive levels of coffee, tea, cola, alcohol, or nicotine?

Social: presence of a new baby, shift work, enuretic child, partner who has nocturia or who snores.

Are you agitated, depressed or anxious and feel 'washed out'?

If you are obese this can be associated with sleep apnoea syndrome.

Deal with the underlying cause, where possible.

Avoid going to bed until you feel sleepy.

Take a warm, milky drink before bedtime.

Regular exercise is helpful, but not just before bedtime.

Relaxation exercises or training (e.g., hypnotherapy) can be helpful; also yoga, meditation, reading, and listening to relaxing music.

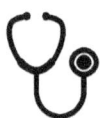 ## UNABLE TO SPEAK

This is a vague symptom. The most common cause is anxiety, but the symptom can also be associated with epilepsy, convulsions, the aftermath of fits, and strokes in adults.

It is also known as mutism, or being mute.

In the past, this was known as selective mutism, associated with anxiety, and very common among young children. It was characterized by the inability to speak in certain situations.

An inability to communicate can occur in children or adults with physical disabilities.

Children with selective mutism communicate only in situations in which they feel comfortable. More than 90% of children are diagnosed with social anxiety. It is common before the age of five years. Some may stand motionless and freeze in specific social settings, and have no communicative ability. Some children may never learn how to speak, causing loss of the speaking ability.

It is also caused by illness in the child or the parents, a neuromuscular problem, or shyness of the child.

Alalia is the term for a delay in the development of speaking abilities in children. Childhood deafness is a major cause.

Anarthria is a severe form of dysarthria which occurs due to problems with the coordination of movements of the mouth, tongue and lungs.

Aphasia is a speech and language problem due to damage of the cerebral centers which deal with language.

Aphonia is the inability to produce any voice. In severe cases, the patient loses phonation. It is caused by the injury, paralysis, and/or illness of the voice box.

Autistic children often don't speak. Many people with autism are also intellectually disabled.

Most intellectually disabled children learn to speak, but in severe cases they can't learn speech.

Down's syndrome children often have impaired language and speech function.

You must consult a doctor if this symptom occurs.

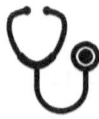

UNCONSCIOUSNESS

WARNING: Never touch a patient who has fainted without checking the surrounding area. Look for cables, wires, urine, faeces, saliva, blood or vomit.

Remember to take care about your well-being. People who have been electrocuted can continue to conduct the electricity through their skin, and blood and vomit can spread infections to others (HIV or Infections).

Treat this as a medical emergency, call 999, and ask for an ambulance to take the patient to hospital.

This symptom refers to the loss of a person's ability to respond to people and activities. This could be described as fainting, a coma, comatose state, or unconsciousness.

This can be linked to, or confused with, a changed mental state (check: altered mental state), confusion, disorientation, delirium or stupor. Major or minor illness or injury, drugs and alcohol may cause this.

Other causes include: the loss of excess fluids, as seen in dehydration due to diarrhoea, vomiting, and severe bleeding (external and internal); low blood sugar levels, resulting from diabetes, metabolic problems, diarrhoea, or vomiting; low blood pressure, possibly related to drugs, vomiting, diarrhoea, or bleeding; low temperature as a result of cold or septic shock; low carbon dioxide as a result of an anxiety attack, rapid breathing, metabolic problems, or hormonal changes; a high temperature as a result of fever, infections, or a head injury; excessive straining during a bowel movement (vasovagal syncope); a vasovagal attack – stimulation of glands in the neck, caused by low blood supply to the brain; coughing very hard; or breathing very fast (hyperventilating).

More rarely, this may be caused by serious heart or nervous system disorders.

This symptom must be differentiated from sleeping: a sleeping person will respond to loud noises, or gentle shaking but an unconscious person will not.

An unconscious patient will not respond to touch, call or other stimuli.

Some other symptoms may occur after a person has been unconscious, which include:

Amnesia concerning events before, during, and even after the period of unconsciousness, confusion, drowsiness, behavioral change, weakness (stupor), a waddling gait and/or unsteadiness, a headache or light-headedness, the inability to move parts of his or her body (stroke/hemiplegia), loss of bowel or bladder control (incontinence), rapid heartbeat (tachycardia, palpitations), inability to speak, difficulty breathing, noisy breathing, high pitched sounds while inhaling, weak, ineffective coughing, or a bluish or pale skin color.

If the person is unconscious from choking, start CPR. Chest compressions may help dislodge the object from the airway.

If you can't feel a pulse or heartbeat, try a firm bang on the chest using the soft part of your fist (the opposite side to your thumb). This can stimulate the heart if the heart is in shock.

After clinical diagnosis, the doctors will often request routine blood tests and investigations to rule out serious causes.

Please also read: "altered state of mind" and "fainting."

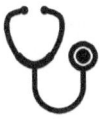 **UNPROTECTED SEX**

There are numerous problems associated with unprotected sex, because the organisms that can spread via genitalia are more numerous than HIV or AIDS. Unlike HIV, these bacteria can be transmitted via genital contact, and oral, anal or penetrating sex.

The most common presentation of an infection is mild and short lived, and so is often not noticed. White discharge and itching in the vagina is often caused by candida – a fungal infection.

A white discharge with no itch is likely to be gonococcus, or another bacterial infection that is transmitted sexually. The discharge may last for a day or two and then disappear, but you will become a carrier and be able to spread the germs to your sexual partner.

If you become pregnant, the child will have serious long-term defects that will be difficult to manage. Blindness, deafness, and congenital heart lesions are common in children of sexually transmitted disease carriers.

If you are a young teenager and have noticed discharge, please go to a GUM or STD clinic. You do not require an appointment, nor will the receptionist question your identity, address, or the name of your GP. You can walk in and get all the tests and treatment free of cost. PLEASE NOTE THAT THIS IS CONFIDENTIAL, and so no one other than the doctors and you will know what disease you have. If you do not want the information shared with your GP, please let the receptionist know.

If the discharge is noticed after unprotected sex, then you must also treat your partner, because he or she will probably have the infection too.

Consult a doctor or a nurse in a GUM or STD clinic in the hospital if the symptoms do not resolve.

You will also need to get tested for other sexually transmitted diseases.

The most common sexually transmitted bacteria that are spreading in the UK and USA are said to have rapidly become resistant to treatment.

One in six women in the USA are said to be infected carriers of herpes genitalia.

PLEASE CONSULT A DOCTOR IN THE GUM CLINIC.

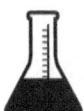 ## URINE – BURNING SENSATION

The common term used by doctors for this symptom is "Dysuria" because of the associated pain when passing urine.

Women often assume this symptom is cystitis, and try to fight the symptom by drinking water, Cranbury juice or electrolyte powders that help change the pH of urine to make it less irritating to vaginal mucosa.

Unfortunately, antibiotic resistant bacteria that do not respond to treatment now threaten us. Reducing delay in establishing the diagnosis and getting treatment early is essential. Please make an appointment with the nurse and get your urine checked early to help reduce future complications.

Please make sure you get your blood pressure checked regularly.

Babies and children may not complain of pain or burning sensations, but will often scream when opening the bowel, or develop constipation.

New-born babies and infants who start to vomit must be investigated for a urinary tract infection, and investigated to rule out congenital abnormalities in the kidney, urinary bladder, and genitalia.

Adults and children may have associated symptoms such as fever, feeling hot and/or cold, behavioral changes, delirium, chills and rigors, increased frequency or inability to pass urine (anuria). You will need a urine culture and microscopy. If blood and proteins are present in urine, the nitrate test is often positive. But if the infection is tested for early, this test may be negative. Please note that this test does not always confirm or rule out the presence of infection, and so must not be relied upon. Patients have developed serious septicaemia because they did not receive the right treatment early.

Please do not waste time before starting treatment if you have all the symptoms that suggest a urinary tract infection, but please make sure you have collected and sent a sample of urine off for testing (microscope and culture sensitivity) in the laboratory.

E.Coli is a common cause of this symptom, and we know the majority of its organisms are resistant to treatment. If symptoms like fever, and pain when passing urine are not better after taking three doses of antibiotics, please consult your doctor and get a urine test.

You must check the lab results before changing the antibiotics or getting admitted to hospital for intra-venous antibiotic treatment.

Please make sure that you get your blood pressure checked regularly.

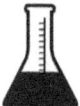
URTICARIAL RASH

Urticaria are small, often itchy, raised red spots, which you can feel. They are rarely serious unless combined with any breathing problems. The rash will usually disappear in a few hours without any treatment. It is most often caused by certain foods and plants (e.g., nettles), but may be caused by a viral infection. A pharmacist may be able to recommend a cream or medicine that could provide some relief. Rarely, the rash may be severe and associated with breathing difficulties: if there is any shortness of breath, dial 999.

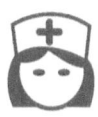

VAGINAL BLEEDING

Blood in urine is seen during a urine infection, or after a traumatic injury of the vagina or penis. This is also the first symptom of a bladder problem, or kidney stones. Normal vaginal bleeding occurs during menstruation, and heavily during abortions. This can be mixed with urine at times. Heavy inter-menstrual bleeding is called dysfunctional urine bleeding (DUB). The most common causes are infections, fibroids in the uterus, or hormonal problems like an over active thyroid. If you are active sexually, and had unprotected sex, please get a pregnancy test.

The bleeding could also be due to retained products of contraception. If the bleeding is profuse and you are passing clots, you may need to go to hospital and consult a gynaecologist. Teenagers or young girls may have started having periods. Pre-pubertal girls with bleeding must be seen by a paediatrician, because this could be traumatic and the child may have psychological problems in the future as a result. Please consult a doctor and go to a GUM or STD clinic if you recently had unprotected sex with a new partner.

VAGINAL PAIN DURING SEX

Pain during or after sex is known as dyspareunia.

Common causes are illness, infection, and a physical or psychological problem.

If you are suffering from this problem, please speak to a doctor. They are used to this and will not be embarrassed.

Pain during sex can affect both men and women.

Tablets like Viagra and others are making sexual intercourse last longer. If the woman is not properly stimulated, the vagina can be dry, and mucosal tears can be traumatic.

Some women are allergic to latex and plastic materials.

Women can experience pain during or after sex, either in the vagina or deeper in the pelvis. Pain in the vagina could be caused by an infection like thrush, chlamydia, gonorrhoea, or genital herpes.

During the menopause, hormone levels can make your vagina dry (vaginitis). Lack of sexual arousal and vaginismus occur because the muscles in or around the vagina shut tightly, making sex painful or impossible.

Genital irritation or allergic reactions can be caused by spermicides, latex condoms, or products such as soap and shampoo.

Pain felt inside the pelvis can be caused by conditions such as: Pelvic inflammatory disease, endometriosis.

See your GP or go to a sexual health GUM (genitourinary medicine) clinic.

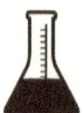 ## VAGINAL THRUSH

Candida albicans is a fungus, which should not normally be present in large numbers in the vagina. For various reasons, it can grow rapidly and cause thrush. Symptoms: A creamy thick white vaginal discharge. Itchiness and irritation. Pain or burning after passing water. Causes are: A prolonged course of antibiotics, the oral contraceptive pill. Hormonal changes preceding the period, Steroid treatment, Diabetes, Immune system problems, Sexual intercourse with an infected man.

Prevention: After being on the toilet, wipe from front to back. Change underwear frequently, particularly after exercise. Choose cotton rather than nylon pants. Avoid harsh soaps; they kill the good bacteria, which prevent thrush.

Complications: There are few serious complications of thrush, but it can, however, make life very miserable. Sex is painful, as is passing water. This fungus has become resistant to treatment, so if the drugs have not helped, please consult a doctor.

Eat live yoghurt and apply it to the vaginal area. It will replace the missing Lactobacillus, which prevents thrush.

Ask your pharmacist for antifungal preparations like miconazole or canesten.

Your partner may need treatment as well.

If the discharge changes in smell or appearance, there is any abdominal pain, or the thrush either does not disappear after self-care or keeps coming back for no apparent reason, please consult your doctor.

See your doctor if the thrush does not disappear after self-care, or keeps coming back for no apparent reason.

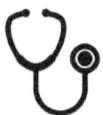 **VERTIGO**

The cause of dizziness in adults and elderly is often vertigo.

This occurs because the nerve in the ears responsible for maintaining our balance is affected.

Feeling dizzy can be very annoying and worrying, but is probably not serious.

If the feeling of dizziness persists, you should certainly be checked out by a doctor.

Feeling dizzy may leave you feeling off balance or lightheaded, or you may feel that everything around you is spinning. You may also hear a weird noise in your ears.

This symptom can be acute or chronic.

Acute, or sudden onset (first time) vertigo needs urgent consultation with a doctor.

If this is chronic, and has happened before, do not panic, but start treatment as before.

The most common causes of dizziness in adults and the elderly are drugs, ear problems, and vertigo. This often occurs because the nerve in the ears responsible to maintain our balance is affected.

Doctor will rule out serious illnesses, and may give anti-sickness pills or antihistamines to reduce the swelling of nerves in the ear.

You may be advised to use steam inhalation, followed by the nasal spray Beconase (Beclomethasone) or Pulmicort (Budesonide) to decongest the sinuses of children and young adults with chronic dizziness.

Serc is a drug often used, but you must be on this treatment for a few weeks.

The diagnosis of this symptom requires proper clinical examination and may require investigation.

Doctors will first check blood pressure, so you must consult as soon as possible.

Shingles in the ear can produce dizziness because the nerve in the ears swells up.

If this symptom is associated with other red symptoms, you must go to hospital now.

If dizziness occurs when you get up out of bed, or stand up from a sitting position, you must speak to a doctor and get your blood pressure and drug treatment reviewed.

If the dizziness that you suffer is sudden, very debilitating, or associated with blurred vision, you must see a doctor.

Please do not drive to hospital but call an ambulance to take you.

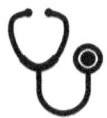 **VISION SUDDEN LOSS OF VISION**

A sudden loss of vision doesn't necessarily mean total blindness.

This symptom can occur in one eye or both eyes, and the loss of sight can be partial or total.

With partial vision loss, some sight may remain in the affected eye.

Sudden loss of vision can be a sudden loss of peripheral or central vision, or even a sudden blurring of your vision.

The sudden appearance of spots or floaters could be more serious.

Sudden blindness may only last a short time, such as a few seconds, minutes or hours. However, it could potentially be permanent, especially if not treated quickly.

Sudden vision loss is very serious, and could potentially be sight threatening or even life threatening. You must consult an eye specialist in hospital, because the retina may be damaged.

The retina is the focusing surface at the back of your eye. This kind of damage is called detachment of the retina. This may cause a total loss of vision in the affected eye, or may only result in partial vision loss, making it seem as if a curtain is blocking part of your vision.

The macula is the central focusing area of the retina at the back of your eye. When a macular hole occurs, it results in a loss of your central vision, while your peripheral or 'side' vision remains.

Vitreous hemorrhages occur when blood leaks within the eye. If this occurs, it can block the light which enters the eye, causing sudden blurred vision, or the sudden appearance of spots within the eye.

There are some serious medical conditions that can cause sudden blindness, such as a stroke or brain tumor. While these causes are quite rare, it is nonetheless important to seek medical attention as soon as possible.

If you experience sudden blindness, or any sudden loss of vision, you need to see an eye specialist straight away. Treatment will depend on the cause of your sudden blindness, but in most cases of sudden blindness, the earlier you are treated, the better your chance of a good outcome.

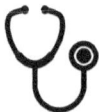 ## VOMITING

The most common cause of vomiting is food poisoning. The key is to differentiate between chemical, bacterial and viral infections. If the vomiting occurs within six hours after consuming some food, it is presumed to be chemical poisoning. Gastritis after alcohol consumption, infections, and also problems in the brain and ears can result in vomiting. Gastro-enteritis is diagnosed if this symptom is associated with diarrhoea. The diagnosis of this symptom requires proper clinical examination, and may require investigation. Doctors will only treat this symptom after ruling out serious illnesses so please consult a DOCTOR. Please do not panic, but go to A&E or the ER if you cannot get an appointment, or you cannot speak to or consult a doctor.

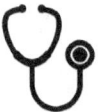 ## VOMITING AFTER BOUT OF COUGH

Vomiting after a severe bout of coughing is typically seen in a child with whooping cough. The child will need a blood test, swab, and treatment. Please consult a doctor. This symptom can occur after a dry cough and coughing in asthmatics. Children on bronchodilators taken via inhaler can have vomiting as a side effect. Poor technique when using an inhaler often causes this problem. Please use a

Volumatic to see if this reduces vomiting. Ask a nurse to check your inhalation technique.

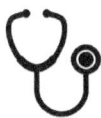 ## VOMITING BLOOD

This symptom is called hematemesis, and the most common cause is gastritis. Diagnosis of this symptom requires proper clinical examination, and may require investigation.

Doctors will only treat this symptom after ruling out serious illnesses, so you must consult a DOCTOR and not a nurse in the UK. Please do not panic, but go to A&E if you cannot get an appointment, or you cannot speak to or consult a doctor.

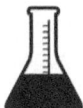 ## WART

Raised pale bumps, or flattened areas with black dots and loops, as though there are some small fibres bundled together are called warts.

This is caused by a virus which is slow growing, so it takes a long time for the body to develop immunity.

Most disappear, but this may take 2–3 years. The body develops immunity slowly, and the lesion disappears as it does.

The common term used is "Viral Wart" and it is a very contagious condition.

There is little evidence to prefer one treatment above another. Of the conventional treatments, salicylic acid appears from the limited evidence available to be the best.

Soak in warm water for 5 minutes twice daily, prior to application of any treatments, rub with a pumice stone or manicure emery paper to remove the outer protective layer of dead skin.

Apply Salactol paint every night for 6–12 weeks. Persevere until the wart has completely disappeared; this may take 3 months.

Cautery is an alternative if the wart is very large.

Use liquid nitrogen – not for children under the age of 10 years, as this can be painful. It can also cause dramatic blood blistering, temporary numbness, and a scar. The procedure can be painful, and has no added value when compared to treatment using silver nitrate (Salactol).

Even vigorous procedures do not always succeed, and warts often reappear at the treated site. A patient with a verruca should use a waterproof plaster or verruca sock for swimming and PE, and avoid sharing a towel.

Children and adults with urogenital warts must be seen by a doctor.

If you are an elderly person with a single wart, please consult a doctor.

Please note that doctors do not have any special treatment or method to cure this wart. Please contact a pharmacist for advice.

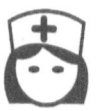 **WEAKNESS**

The diagnosis of this symptom requires proper clinical examination, and may require investigation. The most common cause of this symptom is a transient ischemic attack (TIA), but the problem may be local. Doctors must clinically examine you and advise treatment. Please do not waste time and consult a doctor or demand a home visit. Doctors will not be able to treat this symptom at home. Please do not panic, call an ambulance and go to A&E or the ER if you cannot speak to, or consult a doctor.

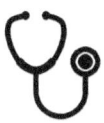

WEAKNESS IN ONE SIDE OF BODY

The diagnosis of this symptom requires proper clinical examination, and may require investigation. The most common cause of this symptom is a transient ischemic attack (TIA), but the problem may be local. Doctors must clinically examine you and advise treatment. Please do not waste time and consult a doctor or demand a home visit. Doctors will not be able to treat this symptom at home. Please do not panic, call an ambulance and go to A&E or the ER.

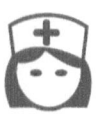

WHEEZING

Apart from asthma, the causes of this symptom are a viral or bacterial infection, anatomical anomalies (including laryngeal problems), an inhaled foreign body, and cystic fibrosis.

Bronchiolitis, caused by respiratory syncytial virus (RSV), can also cause a wheeze.

Parents and doctors in the past labeled, asthma, a recurrent cough, or wheezing as 'wheezy bronchitis', 'wheezy tendency', 'bronchitis', or 'LRTI (lower respiratory tract infections)', and abused antibiotics in consequence.

When attacks of wheezing are brought on by infection, bronchodilators are generally ineffective.

The majority of children and adults diagnosed with 'wheezy bronchitis', are asthmatics unless and until this is ruled out.

Consider asthma in a child with a recurrent cough, especially a nocturnal cough, and in those who are breathless upon exertion.

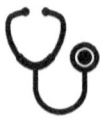 ## WHEEZY COUGH

This cough is usually dry and spasmodic; it occurs in patients suffering from asthma and/or hay fever.

The cough is typically wheezy or musical cough.

People with post nasal drip, or who are smokers often have this cough. The mucus from the sinuses drains down the back of the throat, and the cough caused by this will normally be worse when you lie down, or when you first wake up in the morning.

This is quite common with those who suffer from hay fever, although if an allergy is present that is due to something other than seasonal hay fever, a cough can be present all year round.

Apart from asthma, this cough is associated with some viral and bacterial infections, anatomical anomalies (including laryngeal problems), an inhaled foreign body, and cystic fibrosis.

Bronchiolitis, caused by respiratory syncytial virus (RSV), can also cause a wheeze.

Parents and doctors in the past labeled, asthma, a recurrent cough, or wheezing as 'wheezy bronchitis', 'wheezy tendency', 'bronchitis', or 'LRTI (lower respiratory tract infections)', and abused antibiotics in consequence.

When attacks of wheezing are brought on by infection, bronchodilators are generally ineffective.

The majority of children or adults are diagnosed as having wheezy bronchitis, or bronchitis, and not as asthmatics. Please consult a chest physician, and make sure that you are not an undiagnosed asthmatic abusing antibiotics.

Consider asthma in a child with a recurrent cough, especially a nocturnal cough, and in those who are breathless upon exertion.

Even if you think this is the cause of your morning cough, it is important to have a proper diagnosis made by your doctor.

It is not wise to self-medicate, as many antihistamine preparations will have side effects, and certain type of coughs, like an asthmatic or allergic cough, must not be suppressed.

Asthma inhalers open your airways, and the body will have to get rid of the sputum or phlegm that has collected in the lungs. If the dry cough becomes productive – bringing out lots of phlegm, please do not take cough mixtures or think you have an infection.

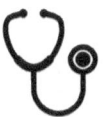

WHITE DISCHARGE FROM GENITALIA

If the discharge is noticed after unprotected sex, you must go to a GUM or STD Clinic and get help.

In the UK, you do not require an appointment but can walk in and get tests and treatment. PLEASE NOTE THAT THIS IS CONFIDENTIAL, and so no one other than the doctor and you know what disease you have.

You will also be tested for other sexually transmitted diseases. It is important to know that the symptoms may resolve without treatment, but you will still be at risk of spreading infection to others, and you may develop complications later. The discharge may be present for one or two days and disappear but the cause will continue to live in your body, and you will pass on the infection to your sexual partners.

Please note that the majority of the bacteria that cause sexually transmitted diseases all over the world are now resistant to treatment.

Delay, or the wrong choice of antibiotics will result in you becoming a carrier, spreading the infection to others, developing long-term complications, and potentially dying.

Early diagnosis and treatment is essential to stop the spread of infections like gonorrhoea, syphilis, chlamydia and genital herpes.

One in six women in the USA are said to be carriers of genital herpes.

PLEASE CONSULT A DOCTOR IN A GUM CLINIC

 ## WHITE DISCHARGE FROM VAGINA

White discharge and itching in the vagina is often caused by candida – a fungal infection.

A white discharge with no itch is likely to be gonococcus, or another bacterial infection that is transmitted sexually. The discharge may last for a day or two and then disappear, but you will become a carrier and be able to spread the germs to your sexual partner.

If you become pregnant, the child will have serious long-term defects that will be difficult to manage. Blindness, deafness, and congenital heart lesions are common in children of sexually transmitted disease carriers.

If you are a young teenager and have noticed discharge, please go to a GUM or STD clinic. You do not require an appointment, nor will the receptionist question your identity, address, or the name of your GP. You can walk in and get all the tests and treatment free of cost. PLEASE NOTE THAT THIS IS CONFIDENTIAL, and so no one other than the doctors and you will know what disease you have. If you do not want the information shared with your GP, please let the receptionist know.

If the discharge is noticed after unprotected sex, then you must also treat your partner, because he or she will probably have the infection too.

Consult a doctor or a nurse in a GUM or STD clinic in the hospital if the symptoms do not resolve.

You will also need to get tested for other sexually transmitted diseases.

The most common sexually transmitted bacteria that are spreading in the UK and USA are said to have rapidly become resistant to treatment.

One in six women in the USA are said to be infected carriers of herpes genitalia.

PLEASE CONSULT A DOCTOR IN THE GUM CLINIC.

 ## WHITE SPOTS IN MOUTH

This is a common symptom in babies who develop thrush.

These babies will often cry and have difficulty feeding, and will often lose weight.

If a child has these white spots, and they are associated with other red symptoms, then the diagnosis is likely to be a viral or bacterial infection that must be adequately treated with the right antibiotics.

If the symptoms or illness do not resolve after taking three doses of antibiotics please consult a doctor.

This is not a common symptom in adults; please consult doctors if you have this symptom. You will be investigated and properly treated with the right drugs if necessary.

Delays in diagnosis can result in complications that can result in long-term illness.

To learn how to manage thrush, please read the notes under "Thrush."

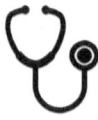 # WHOOPING COUGH

A runny nose, congestion, and fever precede the first stage.

This cough is paroxysmal – including spasms – with possible cyanosis (face going blue to purple), and ending in a whoop. A typical presentation is coughing with a whoop; face going red, and occasionally lips turning blue (cyanosed), and is often associated with vomiting – this is a very useful sign.

Some infants may have no whoop, but present as apnoeic (stopping breathing). This child must be admitted if this symptom is associated, or if there is major distress from the coughing.

Doctors must believe the parents' account of an apnoeic attack – the child may seem well in between coughing fits.

This cough can persist for weeks, or for two to three months.

A blood test helps to confirm diagnosis. A nasal swab is not a practical method of diagnosis.

Please insist on being admitted, or go to a local hospital and consult a paediatrician, because the next apnoeic attack could be fatal.

Admit if the child is under 1 month old. If there is no evidence of respiratory distress, the child can be managed at home.

Some doctors will treat other children at home and prescribe a course of erythromycin. This cough does not respond to conventional cough suppressants, so their use is not advisable.

The incubation period of whooping cough is 7–10 days. The patient is infectious from 2 days prior to the start of symptoms, until up to 5 weeks after the onset of the cough.

Watch the patient's fluid intake, and do not force feed solids if a child refuses them – give them coke, milk or water, symptomatic-tube feeding, oxygen, etc.

Treatment is erythromycin for 14 days.

Non-immune infants and their contacts are said to reduce the infectivity of pertussis (whooping cough). Please note that an immunized child can be infected, but the duration of the illness is reduced.

Complications are cerebral-fits, hemiplegia (like stroke paralysis of one side), encephalopathy in a child under 6 months old, bronchopneumonia, lobar collapse, and death.

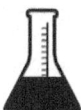 ## WIND OR FLATULENCE

Flatus, wind or gases generated in the stomach or intestine, expelled through the anus is called flatulence, blowing, or breaking wind. Flatus is also the medical word for gas generated in the stomach or bowels.

Intestinal gas may be composed of swallowed environmental air (seen in babies and elderly people with dementia), and hence flatus is not totally generated in the stomach or bowels.

The normal range of volumes of flatus in healthy individuals varies hugely (476–1491 ml/24 h).

Some people complain of belching, burping, abdominal bloating, and discomfort across the abdomen.

Patients with gastro-enteritis, diarrhoea, or on drugs that kill good germs in the stomach, may pass wind and also burp.

Gas is either swallowed environmental air, present intrinsically in foods and beverages, or the result of gut fermentation. This is emitted from the mouth by eructation (burping) and is normal.

Excessive swallowing of environmental air is called aerophobia and is often seen in babies, elderly people with dementia, and seriously ill patients.

Pain, bloating and abdominal distension, excessive flatus volume, excessive flatus smell, and gas incontinence are associated.

Endogenously produced intestinal gases cause 74% of flatus. The volume of gas produced is partially dependent upon the composition of the intestinal bacteria, which is normally very resistant to change, but is also very different in different individuals. The greatest concentration of gut bacteria is in the colon; the small intestine is normally near sterile. Fermentation occurs when unabsorbed food residues arrive in the colon. Therefore diet is the primary factor that dictates the volume of flatus produced.

Reducing undigested fermentable food residues arriving in the colon have been shown to significantly reduce the volume of flatus produced. Abnormal intestinal gas dynamics will create pain, distension and bloating, regardless of whether there is high or low total flatus volume.

Flatulence-producing foods: Beans, lentils, dairy products, onions, garlic, spring onions, leeks, turnips, radishes, potatoes, oats, cashew nuts, wheat, yeast, bread, cauliflower, broccoli, cabbage, brussel sprouts, and foods high in polysaccharide.

Children and adults with lactose intolerance have intestinal bacteria feeding on lactose that increase gas production when milk or lactose-containing substances have been consumed.

High altitude flight and the space program spurred interest in the causes of flatulence: low atmospheric pressure, confined conditions, and stresses peculiar to astronauts were a cause for concern.

The phenomenon of high altitude flatus expulsion was first recorded over two hundred years ago on mountaineering expeditions.

Some worm infestations like giardiasis are also associated with flatulence.

If you are able to go to the toilet and open your bowels, or pass wind (fart) the pain usually goes. If not, a chemist may be able to recommend some medication to ease the pain.

This is a very common problem in women who suffer with chronic abdominal pain, and who are diagnosed as having irritable bowel syndrome (previously called tropical sprue).

Try drinking natural yoghurt, buttermilk, or bio products that contain lactobacillus acidophilus (friendly bacteria). These friendly bacteria will absorb gases and reduce harmful bacteria multiplying in the stomach and so reduce bloating and flatus.

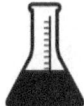

WRIST PAIN

This is a very common symptom that must first be self-treated before consulting a doctor. Doctors will first offer the same treatment that a chemist would advise.

The common treatment is anti-inflammatory analgesics like nurofen, brufen, voltarol, and diclofenac with or without Paracetamol. The main problem with this is gastritis – tummy pain. People with gastritis must consult a doctor.

A doctor will do tests and investigations, and refer you to orthopedics or a rheumatologist if the pain does not resolve with anti-inflammatory drugs.

Please do not stop the treatment as soon as you feel that the pain has gone, but continue for two to three days.

Physiotherapy and exercise when you have pain is not good for you, because the inflamed joint is very brittle and can take more harm. You should exercise or get physiotherapy only after you have taken treatment and the pain has eased.

If you have numbness in your fingers, or chronic wrist pain, please consult a doctor.

Those in professions such as computer programmers or pneumatic drill users often have what is known as RSI and will require help from a doctor.

A tingling sensation in fingers is felt if the ligament in the joints is compressing the nerves and tendons connecting the fingers. This is called Carpal Tunnel Syndrome.